AF730630

10 HERBS EVERYONE SHOULD GROW

By

APRIL D. SPAYD

FDA Disclaimer

Statements made in this book have not been evaluated by the Food and Drug Administration (FDA). Wild Root Farm's information and products are not intended to diagnose, treat, cure, or prevent any disease.

All content is provided for educational purposes only. Herbal products and recommendations are not intended to replace the care of qualified health professionals. Always consult your physician or healthcare provider before beginning any herbal regimen, especially if you are pregnant, nursing, or taking medications.

Dedication

To the plants –
For growing in wild corners, forgotten gardens, and quiet places,
and for offering their medicine to anyone willing to listen.

To the grandmothers, earth workers, and kitchen witches –
Who kept herbal knowledge alive
when the world called it weeds and called you evil.

To my community –
The ones learning, remembering, planting, and passing it on.
This book is for you.

And to my husband –
For your unwavering support, steady encouragement, and belief in me—
even when the garden was overgrown and the dream was still just a seed.
You are my best friend and partner in every root and chapter of this journey.

May your hands stay dirty,
your shelves stay full,
and your tea stay hot.

With roots and gratitude,

April / Wild Root Farm

Welcome to the Garden

You're holding a little piece of Wild Root Farm — a guide rooted in dirt-under-the-nails wisdom and passed-down knowledge. This book was created to help you reconnect with the everyday herbs that have supported wellness across generations. We believe dirty hands make for a happy heart, mind, and soul.

Whether you're tending a backyard plot, a windowsill tray, or a field full of wild ambition, these ten plants offer more than just their leaves. They offer stories, healing, and a deeper relationship with the natural world.

At Wild Root Farm, we believe herbal knowledge should be accessible to everyone. It should be empowering — maybe even a little bit magical. These are the plants we turn to time and again. We trust them to brew tea, balance our systems, ease discomfort, and ground us in nature.

This isn't just a collection of facts. It's an invitation:
To grow your own medicine.
To slow down.
To sip, steep, and savor the moment.

So, pull up a chair. Grab your shears or your teacup.
Let's walk through the garden together — one plant, one tincture, one story at a time.

With roots and gratitude,
Wild Root Farm
Where the WILD grows into medicine.

10 Herbs Everyone Should Grow

Grow your medicine. Know your magic.

Whether you're planting in pots or carving out space in a backyard bed, this guide brings the healing power of herbs into your hands, one plant at a time.

Inside, you'll meet ten essential herbs that are easy to grow, deeply healing, and endlessly versatile, from calming lemon balm to skin-loving calendula. Each plant profile includes practical uses, safety tips, tea rituals, and recipes that turn your garden into a home apothecary.

This is more than a gardening book, it's a return to the roots.

Because when you grow herbs, you grow stories. You grow connection. You grow wild.

"Where the WILD grows into medicine. One plant, one tincture, one story at a time."

Wild Root Farm - www.GrowingWildKY.com

About the Author

April Spayd

April Spayd is the herbalist and heart behind Wild Root Farm in Kentucky, where plants are grown with intention and turned into simple, potent remedies. A lifelong lover of the land, April began her apothecary journey by learning from the wild weeds growing just outside her door.

With muddy boots, ink-stained hands, and a passion for storytelling, she weaves together tradition, intuition, and science to help others rediscover the healing power of plants.

When she's not crafting teas, balms, or teaching others how to grow their own medicine, you'll find her with her hands in the soil, chasing the sun, and thanking the plants that made her who she is.

Unwaveringly supported by her husband, her best friend and biggest believer, this book is a shared dream, rooted in love.

How to Use This Guide

This book was made to be simple, practical, beautiful—and easy to grow with.

Each herb profile includes

- A simple botanical sketch for easy identification
- A clear description of the plant and how to grow it
- Every day herbal uses—from tea to tincture to salve

You can

- Flip to a plant you're curious about
- Use the growing tips to start your own herb patch
- Try a tea, remedy, or recipe
- Build your own seasonal blends or tincture shelf
- Print and display your favorite pages in your apothecary or kitchen
- Take notes at the end of each chapter about what you tried, liked, or would change

Whether you're just getting started or building your family's medicine chest, these 10 herbs are the foundation—trusted, gentle, and powerful.

Start with one plant at a time—and let it teach you.

Herbalism Doesn't Cure—It Helps the Body Remember How to Heal

One of the most common misconceptions about herbalism is that it's a cure-all.
People often ask, "What herb cures anxiety?" or "What tea will fix my skin?" And while we love the curiosity, here's the truth:

Herbalism doesn't cure. It supports.
It restores balance so the body can do what it was designed to do—heal itself.

At Wild Root Farm, that belief is at the root of everything we do.

The Body Is Brilliant

Your body is wise. Constantly recalibrating, it regenerates cells, fights infection, repairs damage, and reaches for harmony.

But life can interrupt that rhythm.
Stress, nutrient-poor diets, chemical exposure, unresolved emotions, and pharmaceutical overload can knock things off balance.
And when they do, you feel it—in your sleep, digestion, mood, energy, and beyond.

That's where herbs come in. Not as cures, but as companions.

What Herbalism Really Does

Herbs work with the body, not against it.
They whisper, remind, and support in ways that are subtle but profound.

They may:

- Calm the nervous system, easing you out of fight-or-flight
- Support detox pathways like the liver and lymph
- Provide minerals and antioxidants to rebuild at the cellular level
- Nourish the gut microbiome, which influences everything from mood to immunity
- Offer grounding, emotional connection, and a sense of ritual

Herbs don't override your body—they encourage it. They help you return to your natural rhythm, step by step.

Not Magic—But Magnificent

This kind of healing is slow. Gentle. Deep.
It's not about instant results; it's about tending over time.
Like a garden—you water, you wait, you trust. And slowly, something blooms.

We're not here to promise miracles.

We're here to offer a partnership—with plants, with your body, with the land.

A way of remembering how to care for yourself that feels ancient and alive.

In a World Full of Quick Fixes, Choose Something Real.

Herbalism isn't a rescue—it's a relationship.
It's not about forcing your body into wellness. It's about working with it, listening to it, trusting it.

So if you're feeling tired, foggy, or disconnected, take heart.
Relief might not come overnight—but it will come.

And the plants will be here when you're ready.

Contents

Why Grow Your Own Herbs?

The Case for Planting Medicine Right outside Your Door

The world is full of quick fixes and store shelves lined with plastic bottles. Growing your own herbs is a quiet act of resistance—a radical return to self-sufficiency. Whether you tend a sprawling plot or a single pot by a sunny window, every leaf you grow is a small reclaiming of your health, your home, and your connection to the natural world.

Here's why it's worth planting your own healing:

1. Freshness and Potency

Herbs lose much of their flavor and medicinal strength during transport and storage. When you grow your own, you harvest at peak potency—when essential oils are most concentrated, colors are deepest, and the plant's life force is most vibrant.

A handful of fresh lemon balm from the garden brews a tea far brighter than anything found in a store-bought bag. And when making tinctures or infused oils, that freshness translates into greater effectiveness.

Your herbs don't just look better—they work better.

2. Self-Sufficiency

Growing herbs is one of the most empowering skills you can cultivate. You're no longer dependent on stores or supply chains for what your body needs.

You can step outside and gather:

- Chamomile for restful sleep
- Calendula for skin healing
- Mint for digestion
- Thyme for colds
- Basil for mental clarity

Whether it's a small ache or a seasonal cold, your garden becomes your first line of care. That's true resilience—grown one leaf at a time.

3. Connection to Nature

Tending herbs slows you down. You start to notice things you once rushed past—like dew beading on lemon balm in the morning or yarrow leaves unfurling like tiny feathers. You might see bees lingering over blooming calendula in the summer sun.

Growing your own medicine fosters presence and reverence. It brings you back into a relationship with the earth—not just as a resource, but as a teacher and partner in your well-being.

Around here, we say, dirty hands make a happy heart. And it turns out, the dirt under your nails may be healing more than your soul.

When you garden, forage, or simply touch the soil, you come into contact with beneficial microbes—like Mycobacterium vaccae—that can:

- Boost your gut microbiome
- Support your immune system
- Improve mood and resilience
- Strengthen your brain–gut connection

Turns out, nature knows what she's doing. The more we connect with the soil, the more we reconnect with ourselves.

So yes—let your hands get dirty. Let your microbes mingle. Let the wild heal you from the outside in. In the garden, healing isn't just what you harvest—it's what you become part of.

4. Cost-Effective Wellness

A packet of seeds might cost a few dollars. A small potted herb, maybe five. But the return is exponential.

From a single plant, you can enjoy:

- Dozens of cups of tea
- Herbs to dry and store
- Materials for salves, oils, and tinctures
- Fresh leaves to cook with—and share

Compare that to store-bought herbal products, often $10–$30 each, and you'll see just how quickly growing your own pays off, season after season.

5. Peace of Mind

When you grow it, you know it.

- You know there are no pesticides or preservatives.
- You know the soil, the sun, and the hands that tended it.

You don't need to decipher labels or question how it was processed—your herbs are whole, alive, and pure.

There's a quiet confidence in that. An emotional ease that comes from knowing you're capable of caring for yourself in a grounded, natural way.

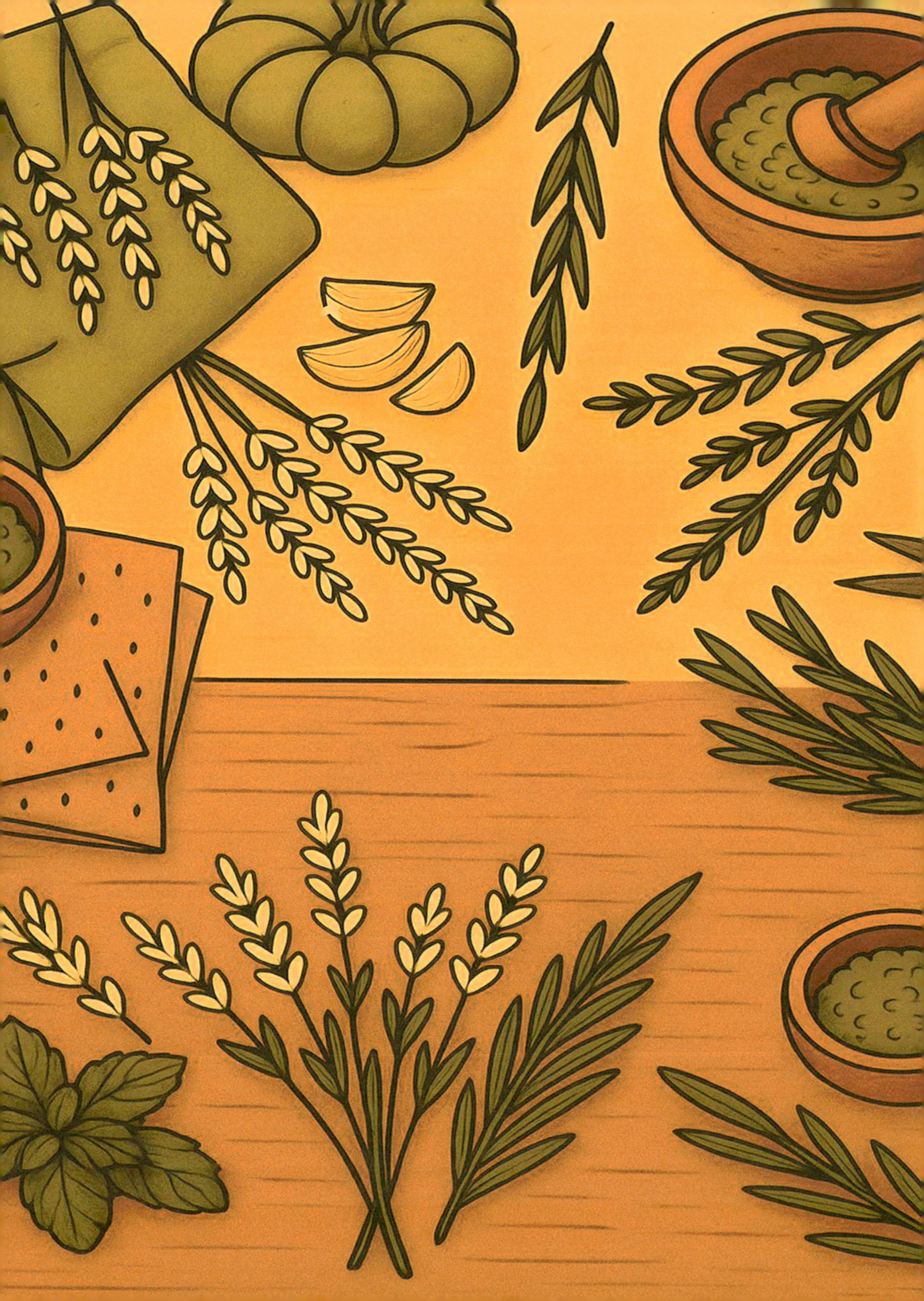

A Final Note from the Garden

Growing herbs isn't just about what you do with them.
It's about who you become along the way.

You become someone who pays attention.
Someone who respects the seasons.
Someone who trusts that healing can be both simple and sacred.

That's what these plants teach.
And that's what this book is here to help you remember.

The Beauty and Purpose of a Home Apothecary

Where Healing Lives on the Shelf and in the Heart

There's something sacred about a shelf lined with glass jars, dried herbs, and handmade remedies. A home apothecary is more than a collection of teas and tinctures—it's a quiet revolution.

It says: I trust the plants. I trust my hands. I trust the slow way.

Whether it lives in a pantry, cabinet, or kitchen corner, your apothecary is where beauty and purpose meet.

A Place of Empowerment

When you steep your own tea or make your own salve, you reclaim something deeply human—the ability to care for yourself and your family.

Your apothecary becomes:

- A remedy for a headache
- A comfort for a child's cough
- A moment of calm after a long day
- A balm for grief, growth, or celebration

It's empowerment in a jar—grown by your hands and guided by nature.

A Space of Beauty

Jars filled with rose petals, calendula blossoms, mint leaves, and calendula buds are more than useful—they're art.

Their colors, textures, and scents stir something ancestral. A memory of medicine made with care.

Labeling each jar, tying bundles with twine, arranging tools in quiet ritual—these are acts of devotion. To yourself. To your craft. To the earth.

It doesn't need to be perfect. It just needs to be yours.

A Resource of Readiness

When colds sweep through, or sleep won't come, your apothecary stands ready. No store runs, no guesswork.

Just a drawer to open, a scoop to pour, a kettle to light.
Your remedies are already waiting—infused with the care and intention you gave them.

A Legacy of Slowness

In a fast world, your apothecary is a slow thing.
It teaches you to sit. To sip. To steep.
To trust the process.
To believe that small, daily acts of care matter.

Each jar, oil, or blend becomes part of a story—of seasons, of stewardship, of healing that unfolds at its own pace.

This is the beauty of herbalism.
This is the purpose of your apothecary.
And this is where your journey begins.

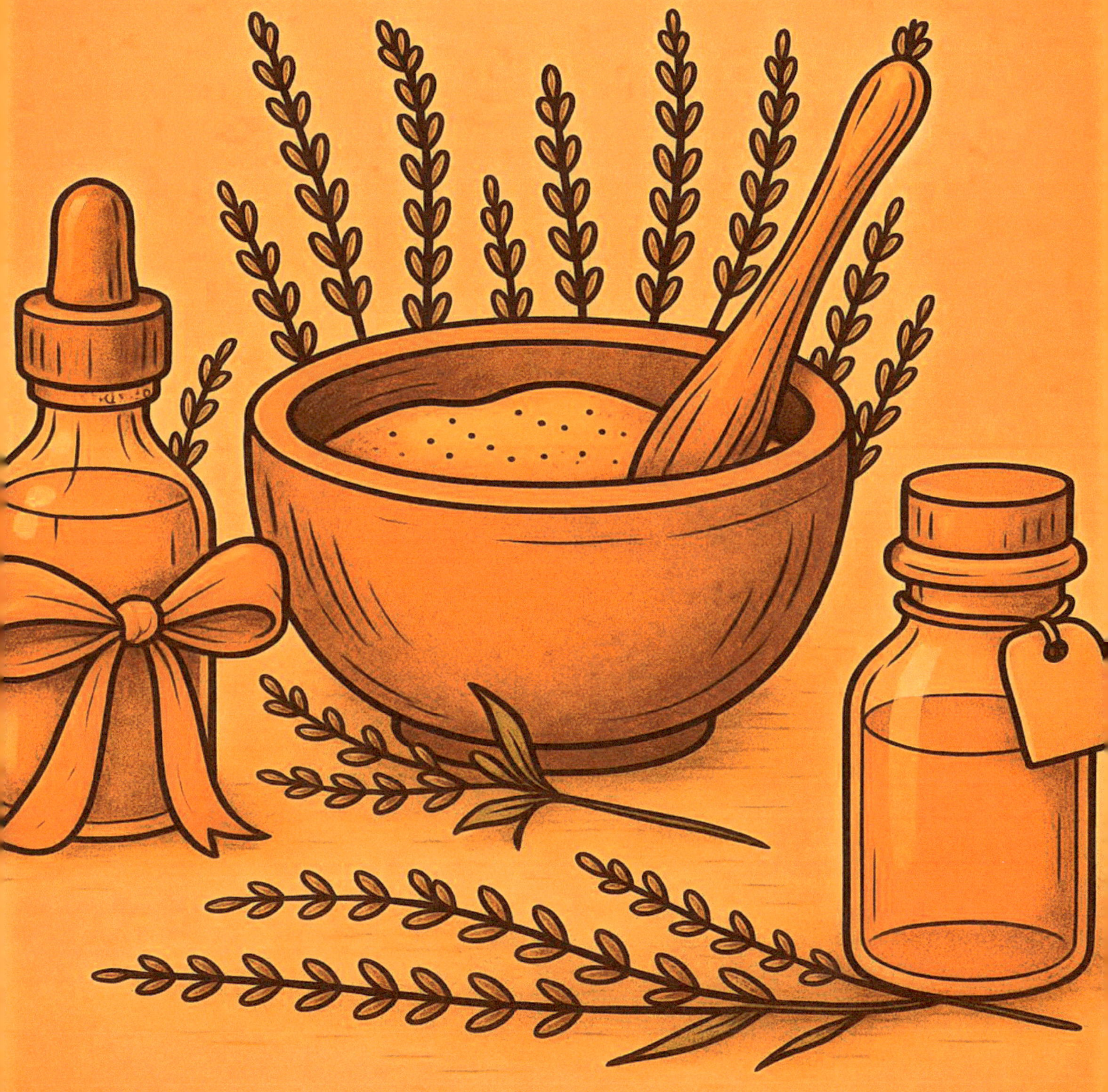

Herbs as Stories and Medicine

More Than Remedies—They Remember for Us

Herbs are more than what they do for the body.
They are stories—living threads woven through generations, lands, and lineages.

Before herbs were bottled or branded, they were carried in grandmothers' hands.
Whispered in kitchens. Picked at dawn. Tucked in pockets "just in case."

- Each plant holds more than its constituents.
- It holds memory.
- It holds meaning.
- It holds medicine—in every sense of the word.

Stories in the Soil

Every herb tells a story:

- Lemon balm hums peace, calming anxious hearts since ancient Greece.
- Calendula remembers wartime wounds, healing skin from Europe to Appalachia.
- Mint recalls kitchens, teas, and summer gardens—forever tied to comfort and clarity.

These plants don't just heal. They connect—to the people who came before, to the wild still growing, and to the parts of ourselves that crave ritual and care.

Medicine That Reminds

Herbal medicine doesn't shout—it whispers.

It reminds us:

- To slow down
- To trust our bodies
- To honor rest as much as action
- That healing isn't always instant—but it is possible

A cup of tea becomes stillness. A poultice becomes prayer.
A tincture becomes a tool for tending—not just the wound, but the whole person.

Personal Practice

Your relationship with each herb becomes its own story. You might remember how chamomile smelled the first time you grew it.

How nettle surprised you with a strength you didn't know you needed.
How chamomile helped you sleep when nothing else could.

This book isn't just a guide. It's a beginning. A seedbed of stories you'll grow into your own.

Let your hands be the next chapter.
Let your garden be your gathering place.
And let each leaf, root, and bloom remind you:

- You are part of something ancient.
- Something healing.
- Something still growing.

Herbal Foundations

Laying the Groundwork for Growing and Using Herbs. Before you plant a single seed or sip your first cup of homemade tea, it helps to understand the heart of herbalism. This isn't about chasing trends. It's about returning to the roots. Herbalism is the art of working with plants to support the body's natural balance. It's slow medicine, seasonal wisdom, and everyday empowerment. In this book, you'll meet ten humble herbs that have stood the test of time. But before we dig into their stories, let's plant a few foundational truths:

The Core Principles of Herbal Practice

Start Small and Learn Deeply

You don't need to grow everything. Begin with one herb.
Learn how it grows. How it tastes. How it feels in your body.

Mastery starts with mindfulness.

Respect the Rhythms

Plants live in rhythm with the earth, the sunlight, the rainfall, the seasons, the soil. The more you observe, the more you'll understand.

Let your garden be your teacher.

Use What You Grow

Herbalism is hands-on. Drink your tea. Infuse your oils. Make a salve.
Each harvest is an invitation to connect with the medicine you've grown.

Start simple. Learn as you go.

Safety Matters

Even gentle herbs deserve respect.
Know how and when to use them—especially with children, elders, or alongside medications.

When in doubt, research and consult.

Let Healing Be Simple

Herbalism isn't about complexity.
It's about supporting the body's natural ability to restore itself.
One plant can offer dozens of gifts.

You don't need to overdo it.

The Wild Root Way

I believe herbal knowledge should be accessible, practical, and personal. This book is your invitation to start small, grow wild, and remember—healing begins in your own backyard.

Choosing Your Own Garden Space

Start Where You Are, Grow What You Can

You don't need acres of land or perfect soil to grow healing plants.
You need sunlight, intention, and a willingness to begin.
Your herb garden can be as small as a windowsill box or as wide as a meadow.
What matters most is that it's yours.
This is about choosing a space that fits your life—not someone else's idea of what a garden should look like.

Light Is Life

The most essential ingredient? ***Sunlight.***
Most herbs thrive with at least 6 hours of full sun each day.
Not sure if your space qualifies? Watch it for a few days.
Where does the light fall in the morning?
What stays brightest through the afternoon?

Even a south-facing balcony, porch railing, or kitchen window can host a small but mighty medicine garden.

Soil Matters—*But* You Can Build It

Herbs prefer well-drained, slightly sandy soil with good airflow around the roots.
But don't let poor soil stop you. You have options:

- **Raised beds:** Great for control and accessibility
- **Containers and pots:** Ideal for patios or mobile setups
- **In-ground rows:** Perfect if you've got space and long-term plans
- **Repurposed spaces:** Old wheelbarrows, crates—even bathtubs—can become herb havens

Wherever you plant, enrich the soil with compost or organic matter if it feels heavy or depleted.
Healthy soil = healthy medicine.

Think like a Plant

- Each herb has its own temperament.
- Some sprawl (like mint), others grow tall (like calendula).
- Some prefer dry roots (like rosemary); others thrive with moisture (like lemon balm).

Group plants with similar needs together. And ask yourself:

- Will this spot get too hot in the afternoon?
- Does water collect here after rain?
- Will I remember to water pots on the porch?

Plants thrive when we treat their needs like relationships—not chores.

Proximity Builds Practice

- Keep your herbs where you'll see them.
- A pot near the back steps gets watered more often.
- A cluster outside the kitchen encourages you to pluck fresh leaves for tea or dinner.
- The more visible and accessible your plants are, the more likely you are to use them, care for them, and grow your confidence.

Beauty Counts, Too

- Choose a space that feels good to be in - somewhere that invites you to linger.
- Add a bench. A stone path. A wind chime or two. Let it be your sanctuary—not just a utility space.
- This is where your medicine begins.
- It should feel like home.

The Wild Root Way

I believe the best garden is the one you actually use.
Not perfect. Not Pinterest-ready. Just possible.
Because healing doesn't need perfection.
It needs presence.

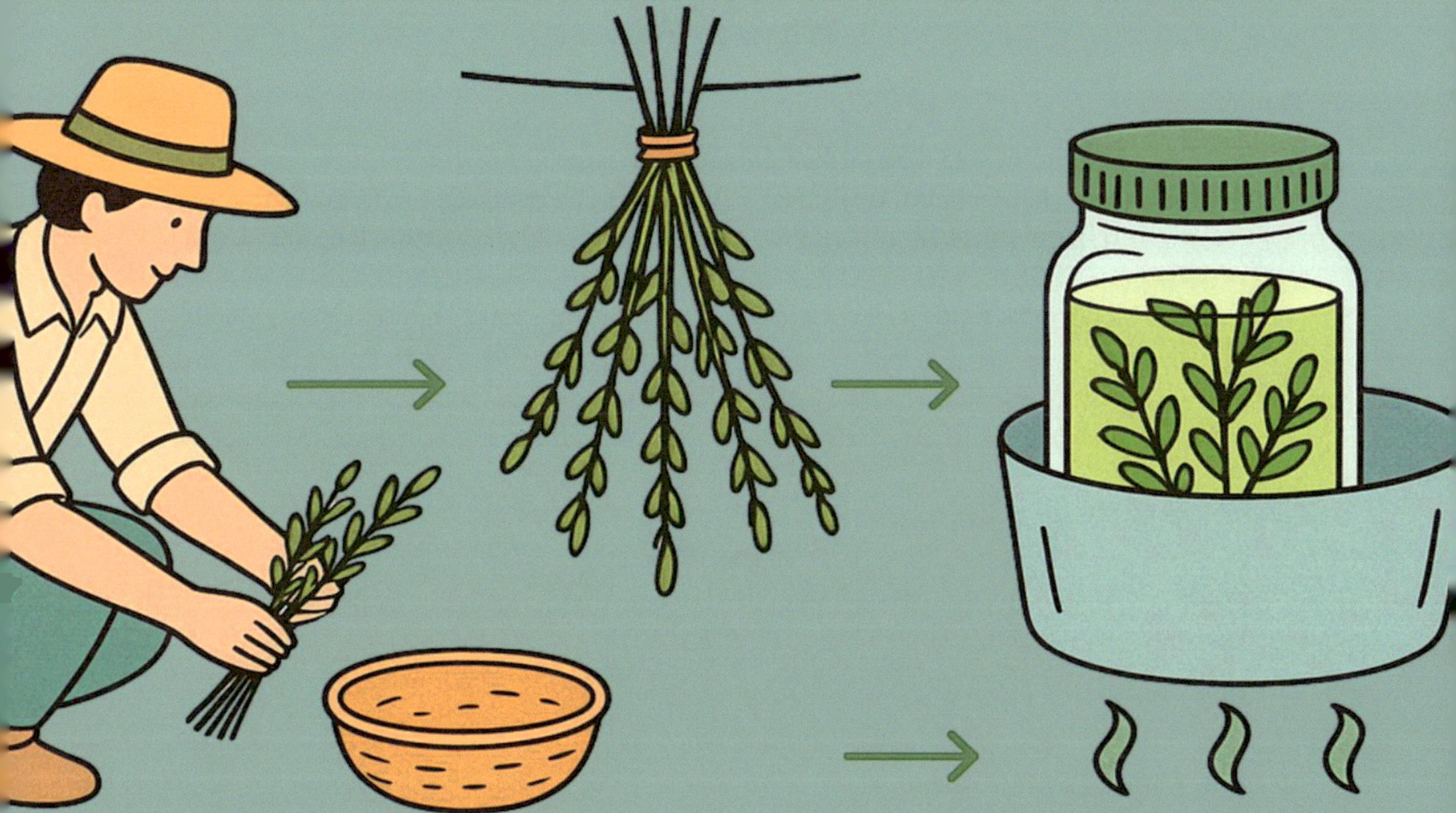

Garden Notes

Preserving the Gifts of the Garden

Tending herbs is only half the journey. How you harvest, dry, and store them determines their potency—and how healing they will be when you need them most.

Think of this process as a quiet conversation with the plant - *You've grown me with care. Now harvest me with honor. Preserve me with love.*

Each leaf, flower, and root has its own season and rhythm.

When you learn to listen, you'll gather more than medicine.

You'll gather memory, ritual, and skill.

When to Harvest

Timing matters

Different parts of the plant hold their medicine at different stages:

- Leaves **(mint, lemon balm, tulsi):** Harvest before the plant flowers—when oils are strongest
- Flowers **(chamomile, calendula):** Pick just as they open. If you wait too long, they begin to lose strength
- Roots **(echinacea, nettle):** Harvest in fall, when the plant's energy returns below ground

Always harvest in the ***morning***, after the dew has dried but before the sun draws out essential oils. Use clean, sharp scissors, shears, or your hands—never tear. And never take more than the plant can spare.

How to Dry

Drying preserves your herbs well beyond the growing season.
Done right, it maintains potency, color, and aroma. Done wrong, you risk mold or loss of medicinal strength.

Air Drying (Best for Most Herbs)

- Bundle small bunches with twine
- Hang upside down in a dry, shaded, well-ventilated space
- Avoid direct sunlight—it fades the color and weakens the medicine
- Thin leaves dry in 3–7 days; thicker stems or blooms may take up to 2 weeks

Screen Drying

- Spread herbs on a mesh screen or basket
- Ideal for petals and delicate herbs like chamomile or lemon balm
- Flip occasionally to ensure even drying

Dehydrator Drying

- Use only on the lowest heat setting (~95°F)
- Great for humid climates or larger harvests
- Avoid oven drying—the heat is too high and can cook the herbs instead

How to tell when herbs are dry:

- They should be crisp and crumble easily.
- If they bend or feel soft, they need more time.

How to Store

Store your dried herbs like they're precious—because they are.

- Use glass jars with tight-fitting lids (mason jars, amber glass, or recycled spice jars work well)
- Always label with name and date
- Store in a cool, dark place—away from heat, humidity, and light
- Avoid plastic bags or clear containers unless kept inside a dark cabinet

Most dried herbs are best used within 6–12 months for peak potency. However, roots, barks, and some seeds can last longer when stored properly.

A Note on Respect

Harvesting is not just about technique. It's about a relationship.

Thank your plants.
Harvest with mindfulness.
Leave enough for the bees, the soil, and next year's seed.

When you dry and store herbs with intention, you're creating more than a pantry.
You're building a medicine cabinet—one that holds summer's sunlight, spring's energy, and autumn's wisdom, all preserved in jars.

Ready for the months ahead.
Ready when needed.

I believe the harvest is holy.
It's the bridge between plant and practice, between garden and healing.

Gratitude

To the plants
who rise each day from seed and root,
offering fragrance, flavor, healing, and truth.
We thank you for your medicine,
your grace, your green wisdom.

To the land
that cradles the roots and holds our steps,
where wild things grow and stories are kept.
We honor your ancient memory
and the life you nurture so patiently.

To the sun
golden keeper of warmth and bloom,
who stirs the leaves and lifts the gloom.
With every beam, you give us light
and kindle hope from morning to night.

To the pollinators
wings humming through herb and vine,
bridging life one bloom at a time.
To bees, moths, birds in sacred flight,
we bless your dance, your work, your rite.

To the circle of souls
the elders, the teachers, the hands now gone,
who whispered the wisdom we carry on.
To kindred hearts and spirits near,
we feel your presence, ever clear.

To the Creator
breath of stars, source of seed,
we praise the pulse behind each need.
In every petal, stone, and sky,
your love endures, your truths reply.

May we walk gently, gather wisely, and grow in harmony with all that gives freely.

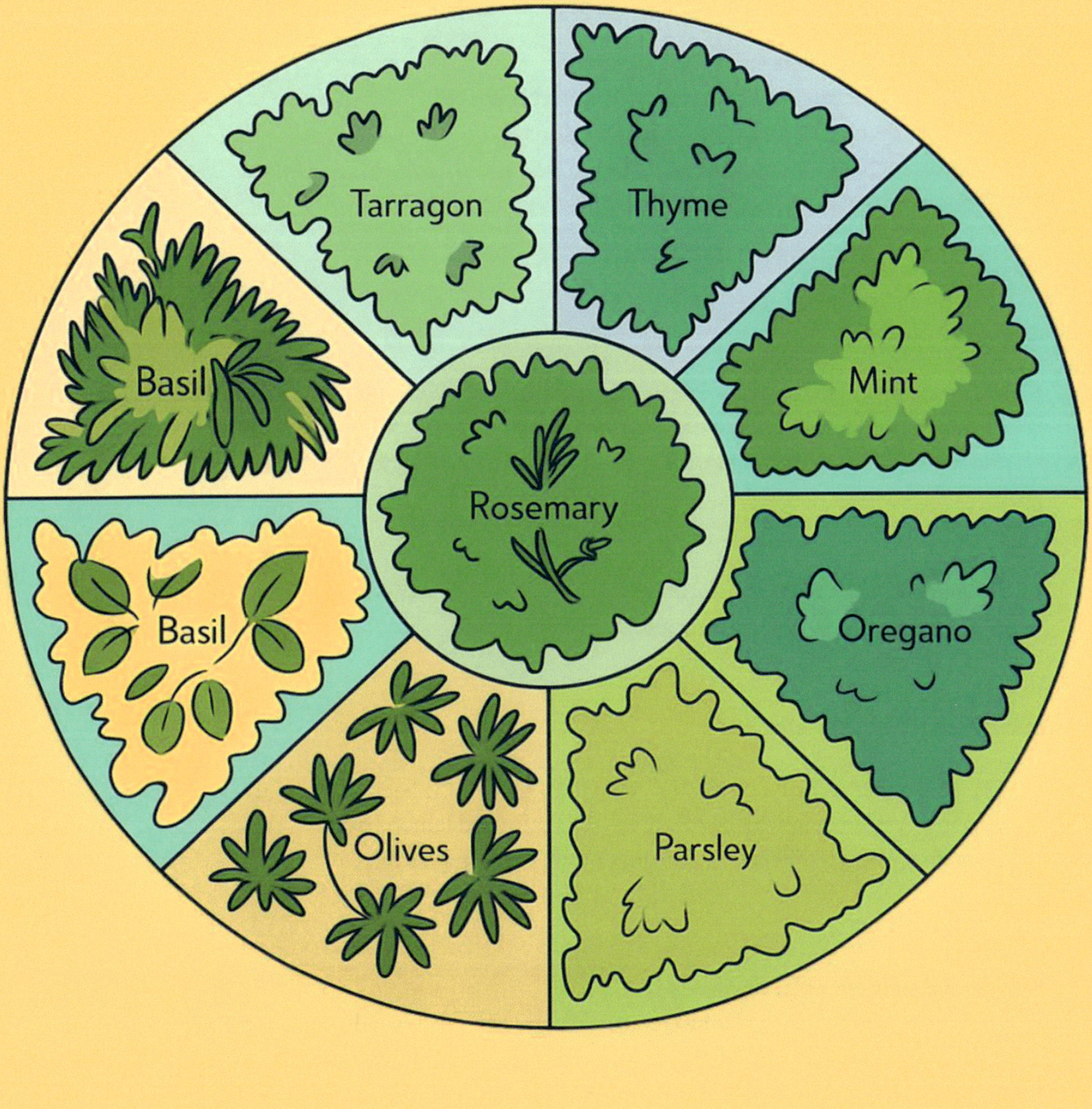
Tarragon
Thyme
Basil
Mint
Rosemary
Basil
Oregano
Olives
Parsley

How to Create a Small Kitchen Garden Medicine Wheel

Grow your remedies within reach, right outside your door

A medicine wheel garden isn't just practical, it's symbolic. Each herb takes its place in the circle, reflecting the balance between nature and body.

In just a few feet of space, you can grow a powerful apothecary of flavor, healing, and beauty.

What you'll need:

- A sunny spot near your kitchen or back door
- 10 medicinal herbs (like the ones featured in this book)
- Stones or dividers to mark the circular sections
- Compost-rich soil or a raised garden bed
  (Optional): A center stone, stepping stones, and plant labels

Step-by-Step Instructions

Design Your Circle

- Choose a space of about 2-4 feet in diameter
- Use rope, wood, or stones to divide it into 8–10 wedge-shaped segments (like slices of pie)
- Place a small stone or meaningful object in the center to symbolize grounding.

Prepare the Soil

- Loosen soil to a depth of 8–12 inches.
- Mix in compost or well-rotted manure for fertility.
- Make sure the area has good drainage.

Plant by Properties or Aesthetics

- Place taller herbs (like rosemary or echinacea) toward the back or the north-facing edge
- Group complementary herbs together—like mint and lemon balm
- Contain spreaders (like mint) with pots or underground barriers

Water and Mulch

- Water deeply after planting.
- Add mulch around each plant to retain moisture, suppress weeds, and nurture the soil.

Harvest with Care

- Snip leaves or flowers as needed using clean, sharp scissors.
- Always leave enough for the plant to regenerate.
- Use fresh or dry for teas, tinctures, and remedies.

Why It Works

- The circular shape reflects nature's cycles, harmony, and seasonal flow
- Small-space friendly—perfect for patios, porches, or raised beds
- Deeply symbolic—each herb brings medicine, memory, and meaning

Plant your intentions. Harvest your healing.
Let your garden become a wheel of wisdom, rooted in ritual and bloom.

The Plant Companions

Ten Herbs to Grow, Know, and Love

These ten herbs are more than entries in a guide—they're allies. Teachers. Friends. Each one brings its own story, energy, and medicine. Each one has something to offer your body, your garden, and your spirit. Some soothe the nervous system, while some strengthen digestion. Some brighten your mood or help you sleep easily.

They are trusted, time-tested, and gentle enough for everyday use.
You don't need to memorize everything.
Start with one. Spend time with it. Grow it. Sip it. Listen.
Let it teach you, one leaf and one experience at a time.

Lemon Balm

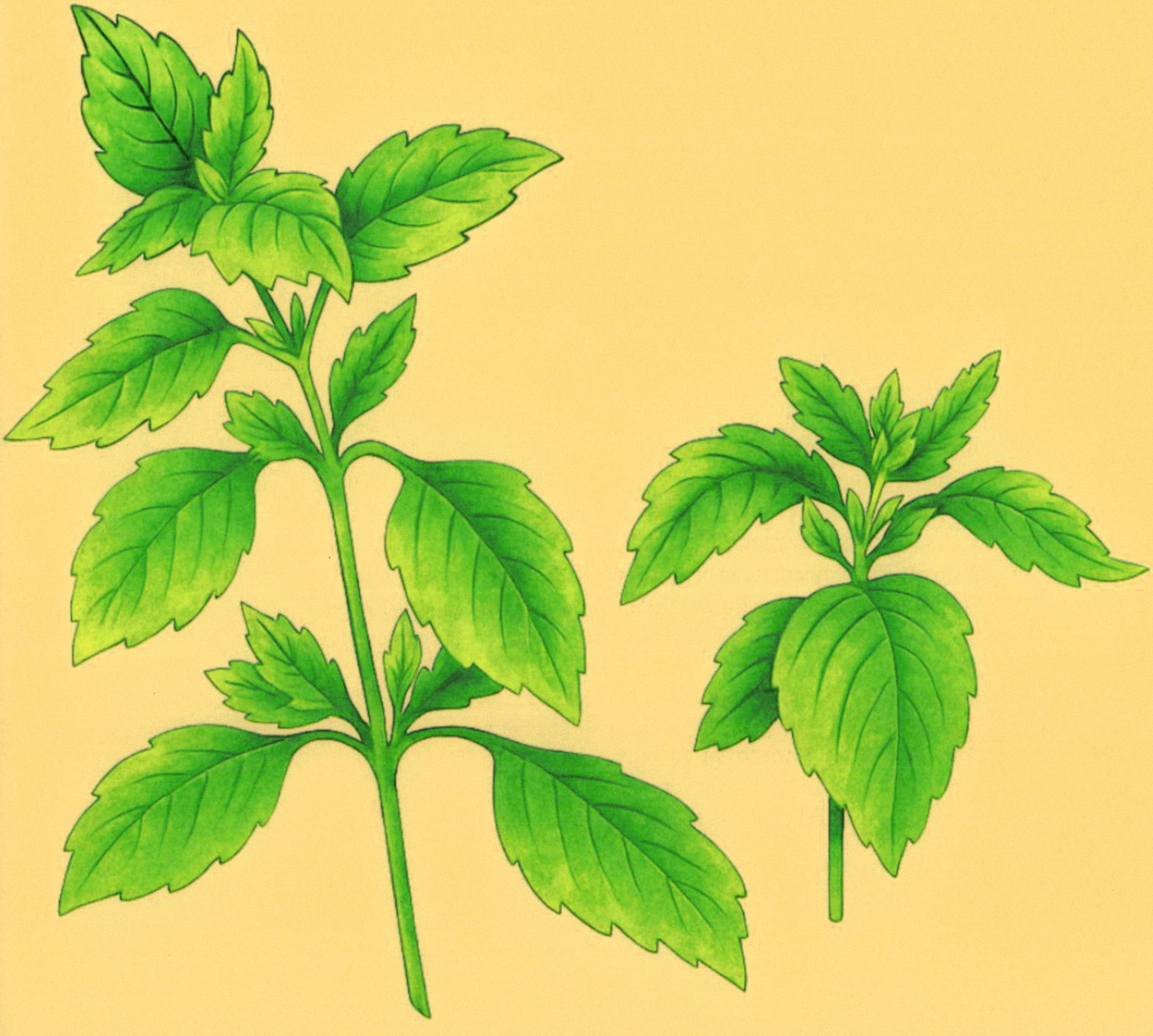

Lemon Balm (Melissa officinalis)

Why Grow It?

Lemon balm eases anxiety, lifts mood, and supports restful sleep. It's a gentle antiviral and makes a delicious tea or tincture.

Plant Profile

- **Botanical Name**: Melissa officinalis
- **Common Names**: Bee balm, sweet balm, heart's delight
- **Family**: Lamiaceae (Mint family)
- **Parts Used**: Aerial parts (leaves and flowering tops)
- **Taste**: Sweet, citrus-y, slightly tart
- **Energetics**: Cooling, slightly drying
- **Actions**: Nervine, carminative, antiviral, mood-lifting, mild sedative

Botanical Description

When crushed, the leaves release a bright, lemony scent that soothes both body and spirit.

Grow Tip: It spreads easily; consider container growing. Cut back regularly to encourage fresh growth.

Medicinal Uses

1. Nervous System Support

- Reduces anxiety, tension, and irritability
- Soothes panic, restlessness, and racing thoughts
- Supports focus for ADHD and scattered energy
- Eases emotional heaviness, grief, and seasonal sadness
- A dropperful of tincture can uplift the mood during emotional lows
- Steep 1 tbsp fresh leaves (or 1–2 tsp dried) in hot water for 10–15 minutes
- Pairs well with holy basil or St. John's wort (use caution with interactions)

2. Herbal Steam for Tension Relief

- Add a handful of leaves to hot water
- Inhale gently with a towel over your head
- Helps ease tension headaches and sinus pressure

3. Digestive Aid

- Relieves bloating, gas, and stress-related cramping
- Calms nervous digestion
- Drink as tea or take a tincture after meals
- Combine with mint or fennel for added support

4. Antiviral & Immune Support

- Especially effective against herpes simplex (cold sores)
- Used both topically and internally for colds, flu, and viral flares

5. Sleep & Calm

- Eases insomnia linked to stress or circular thoughts
- Gently sedates without grogginess
- Safe for children and elders as a bedtime tea
- Blend with chamomile and lavender for a soothing nighttime infusion

6. Cold Sore Relief (Topical)

- Infuse leaves in olive oil or brew a strong tea
- Dab directly on cold sores to soothe irritation and speed healing

7. Bug Bite Soothe Spray

- Brew strong lemon balm tea, let cool, and transfer to a spray bottle
- Apply to bug bites, mild rashes, or sun-irritated skin

Culinary Infusion

- Chop fresh lemon balm into fruit salads, lemonades, or vinegars
- Delicious with strawberries, cucumbers, and honey
- Try a lemon balm + strawberry shrub for a bright, tangy tonic

Traditional & Folk Uses

- Used by Hildegard of Bingen for "melancholy and heartbreak"
- A staple in medieval monastic gardens
- Believed to bring joy, clarity, and long life

Magical & Energetic Associations

- **Element:** Water & Air
- **Planet:** Moon & Jupiter
- **Chakras:** Heart and Solar Plexus
  - — Used for joy, healing, clarity, dream work, and peace
  - — Attracts bees, soothes grief, and invites emotional balance

How to Use Lemon Balm

Infusion (Tea)

- 1–2 tsp dried leaves per cup of water
- Steep 10–15 minutes, covered
- Drink for digestion, calm, and lymphatic support

Tincture

- Fresh or dried in alcohol (1:2 or 1:5)
- Dose: ½–1 tsp up to 3x/day

Oil Infusion / Salve

- Infuse dried leaves in olive or jojoba oil for 2–6 weeks
- Strain and use as-is or combine into a calming balm

Aromatherapy & Steam

- Crush fresh leaves and inhale
- Or make a steam bowl to lift mood and ease congestion

Infused Honey

- Layer fresh leaves in a jar, cover with raw honey
- Let infuse 1–2 weeks
- Use in tea, on biscuits, or by the spoonful for sore throat and anxiety

Lemon balm is where joy meets gentleness. It's a reminder that healing can be bright, fragrant, and beautifully simple.

How to Grow Lemon Balm

Cooling. Citrus-scented. Calming.

Lemon balm (Melissa officinalis) is one of the easiest and most rewarding herbs to grow. A perennial in the mint family, it's beloved for its uplifting aroma, gentle action on the nervous system, and endless uses in teas, tinctures, skincare, and pollinator gardens.

1. Growing from a Nursery Start (The Easiest Way)

Buying a small potted plant from your local nursery is the fastest way to get started.

When to Plant
Late spring, once all danger of frost has passed.

Where to Plant

- **In the Ground:** Choose a spot with full sun to partial shade. In hot climates, afternoon shade helps prevent leaf scorch. Lemon balm spreads vigorously—consider using a root barrier, or dedicate a space where it can roam.
- **In a Container:** Highly recommended to control spreading. Use a pot at least 8–12" in diameter with drainage holes. Perfect for patios and kitchen gardens.

Soil - Prefers moist, fertile, well-drained soil. Amend sandy or clay-heavy soil with compost.

Watering - Water deeply after planting. Keep soil evenly moist, especially during dry spells.

2. Growing from Cuttings (Easy & Free)

Lemon balm roots easily from cuttings—ideal for propagation or sharing.

When to Take Cuttings?
Late spring to early summer during active growth.

How to Propagate?

- Select a healthy, non-flowering stem (2–4 inches long).
- Remove lower leaves, keeping 2–3 leaves at the top.
- *Option 1:* Place in a glass of water with leaf nodes submerged. Change water every few days. Roots form in 1–2 weeks.
- *Option 2:* Insert directly into moist potting soil. Gently firm soil around the stem.

Transplanting: When roots are about 1 inch long (or you feel resistance in soil), transplant into a pot or garden bed.

3. Dividing Mature Plants (Instant Results)

If you have an established lemon balm, you can divide it into multiple plants.

When to Divide

Early spring (before growth starts) or fall (after the season slows).

How to Divide

- Gently dig up the plant.
- Separate the root ball into smaller clumps, ensuring each has roots and shoots.
- Replant divisions immediately, using the same planting tips above.

4. Growing from Seed (Slower but Satisfying)

When to Sow

- Indoors: 6–8 weeks before last frost (March–May)
- Outdoors (Direct Sow): After frost, when soil is warm

Sowing Tips

- Lemon balm seeds need light to germinate—do not bury deeply.
- Sprinkle seeds on moist soil and press lightly for contact.
- Cover with a thin layer of vermiculite if desired.
- Keep moist and warm (use a humidity dome or plastic cover if indoors).
- Germination: 10–20 days.

Thinning/Transplanting

Thin or transplant seedlings when they develop a few true leaves. Space 18–24 inches apart in garden beds.

General Care & Maintenance

- **Sunlight** - Full sun to partial shade (4–6 hours of sunlight minimum).
- **Watering** - Consistent moisture, especially for young plants. Mature lemon balm is somewhat drought-tolerant but thrives with regular watering.
- **Fertilizing** - Not a heavy feeder. Top-dress with compost annually or use a light organic fertilizer. Too much fertilizer may dilute the plant's aromatic oils.

Pruning & Harvesting

- Regular leaf harvesting encourages bushier growth
- Cut flower stalks promptly to preserve leaf quality and prevent reseeding
- Mid-summer, trim back by one-third for a flush of new, aromatic growth

Lemon Balm Is Resilient

Whether you're starting with seeds, cuttings, or a nursery plant—lemon balm will reward you with bright leaves, calming energy, and endless uses in your herbal toolkit. Just give it decent light, moist soil, and occasional care, and it will thrive beautifully.

Seed Starting Guide

How to Sprout Lemon Balm

You'll Need

- Lemon balm seeds
- Seed-starting mix (light, well-draining)
- Seed trays or small pots
- Spray bottle or gentle watering can
- Sunny windowsill or grow light

Steps

1. Moisten the seed-starting mix before sowing.
2. Sprinkle seeds on the surface—press lightly. Do not bury.
3. Cover tray with a humidity dome or plastic wrap.
4. Place in a warm, bright spot. Mist daily to keep surface moist.
5. Once seedlings emerge, remove dome and provide good airflow.
6. Transplant when seedlings have at least 2 sets of true leaves.

Step-by-Step: How to Grow Lemon Balm from Seed

Start Indoors

Begin 6–8 weeks before your last frost date.

1. **Prepare the Trays**
   Fill seed trays with moist seed-starting mix. Lightly press it to firm—not too tightly.
2. **Surface Sow Seeds**
   Sprinkle seeds on top of the soil. Do not cover them deeply—lemon balm needs light to germinate.

3. **Mist Gently**
   Use a spray bottle to keep the surface moist but not soggy.
4. **Provide Warmth and Light**
   Ideal germination temperature: 65–75°F (18–24°C). Place in a sunny window or under grow lights.
5. **Be Patient**
   Germination takes 10–21 days. Some seeds may sprout earlier than others—slow but steady!
6. **Thin or Transplant**
   Once seedlings have 2 sets of true leaves, thin them or transplant to larger pots or garden beds.

After Sprouting: Transplanting Tips

- Harden off seedlings gradually before planting outside.
- Space them 12–18 inches apart in a spot with sun to partial shade.
- Water regularly, but avoid waterlogged soil.

Can You Eat Lemon Balm Sprouts?

Technically, yes—they're not toxic, but they're not typically eaten as microgreens.

- **They grow slowly**
- **Their lemony flavor** is best enjoyed when fully grown
- **Better as a calming herbal remedy** for tea, tinctures, or oils

Summary: Sprouting Lemon Balm

- Easy to grow from seed
- Slow to germinate—give it 2–3 weeks
- Needs light to germinate—do not bury the seeds
- Worth it for long-term use in teas, oils, syrups, and skincare

Lemon Balm Herbal Tea Sipping Chart

Form	Amount per 8oz water	Steeping Time	Best for
Fresh leaves	1–2 tablespoons (chopped)	10–15 minutes	Gentle flavor, daily sipping, summer brews
Dried leaves	1–2 teaspoons	10–15 minutes	Stronger medicinal effect, winter use
Strong infusion	¼ cup dried or ½ fresh	30–60 minutes (covered)	Deeper calming, digestive or cold support
Cold brew	2 tbsp fresh or 1 tbsp dried	Steep 4–8 hours in cool water	Refreshing, lightly calming, kids' tea

- Always cover your tea while it steeps to preserve volatile oils like rosmarinic acid (important for calming effects).
- Strain and enjoy warm or iced. Sweeten with honey or lemon if desired.
- Store extra in the fridge for up to 24 hours.
- Great before bed or during stressful afternoons.

Safety of Lemon Balm by Age Group

Infants (Under 1 Year)

- Use with caution and only externally (e.g., mild herbal baths).
- Internally, avoid unless under professional guidance due to sensitive systems.

Children (1–12 Years)

Generally safe in low doses, such as:

- Mild tea (1–2 tsp per cup, steeped briefly)
- Glycerite or diluted tincture (alcohol-free if possible)

Herbal baths or bug bite sprays

- Great for calming nervous energy, stomachaches, and bedtime routines.
- Commonly used in calming blends with chamomile and catnip.

Teens & Adults

- Very safe in tea, tincture, infusion, or as food.
- Excellent for stress, digestion, sleep, and mood enhancement.

Elderly

- Safe and beneficial for mild cognitive fog, anxiety, and digestive discomfort.
- May help with memory issues or early dementia (some studies show benefits in Alzheimer's support).

When to Use Caution

- **Thyroid Disorders:** High doses or long-term use may interfere with thyroid hormones. Consult a healthcare provider if on thyroid medication.
- **Pregnancy:** Generally safe in moderate culinary/tea amounts. Strong tinctures or long-term use should be avoided unless advised by a practitioner.
- **Allergies:** Rare, but if allergic to other mint-family herbs (Lamiaceae), test cautiously before use.

LEMON BALM NOTES

Personal Experiences

Preparations Tried

Favorite Uses

Blends / Parings

Harvest Notes

Other thoughts

Lemon Balm: The Queen's Forgotten Garden

Long ago, there was a queen who ruled a prosperous land, yet carried a heavy heart. Her castle was filled with gold, music, and splendor, but grief clung to her like a shadow. She had lost her beloved sister during a harsh winter, and since that day, the queen no longer smiled. The once-lush gardens of her palace wilted from neglect.

One morning, an old gardener woman arrived at the castle gates, carrying a basket of herbs and the sweet whisper of honey in the air.

"I have nothing to give but comfort," the woman said, "and this little leaf, if you'll let it grow."

She pressed into the queen's hand a sprig of green—a small, heart-shaped leaf with the scent of lemon and sunshine.

The queen planted it in the forgotten garden. Days passed, and the herb grew quickly, its fragrance drifting through the palace windows. Bees began to return, dancing in the warm air. As the queen walked among the leaves, breathing in their sweet scent, her heart began to soften.

She made tea from the leaves, and for the first time in years, she slept peacefully.

As the seasons turned, the queen smiled again. She reopened the gardens to the people and named the herb Melissa, meaning "honeybee," in honor of its gift: a gentle lifting of sorrow, a return of joy, and the healing hum of life continuing.

The Legacy of Lemon Balm

- Planted near homes to invite happiness and drive away melancholy
- Carried in charm bags to ease anxiety and mend broken hearts
- Infused in teas for sleep, peace, and emotional healing
- Believed to attract bees, blessings, and beloved spirits

Lemon balm reminds us that even the heaviest grief can be soothed with time, sweetness, and the soft hum of something living returning to bloom.

Calendula

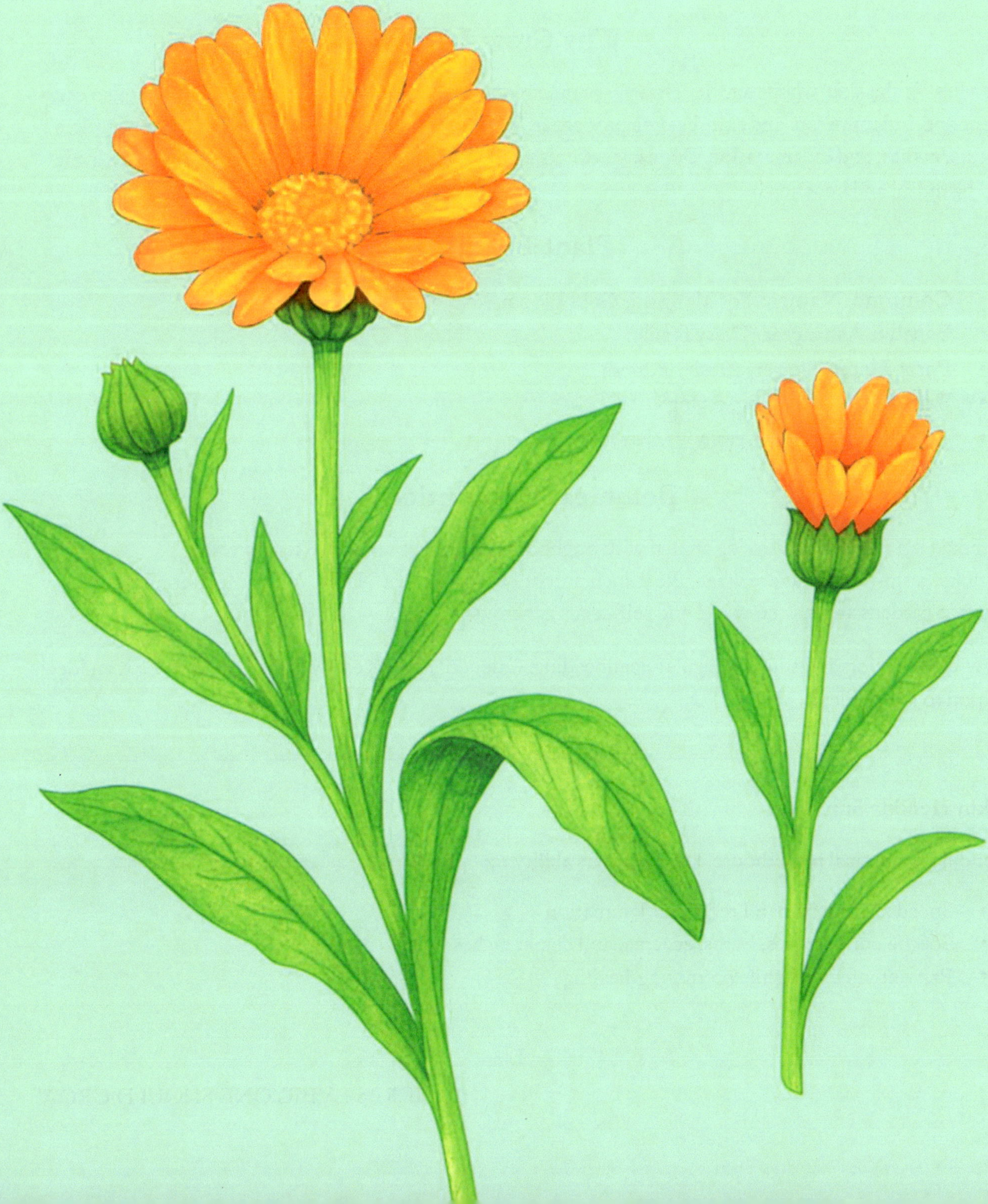

Calendula (Calendula officinalis)

As we explore these herbs, we're not just cultivating a garden of medicine. We're cultivating a deeper connection with the natural world, a space where healing happens slowly, in harmony with the seasons and cycles. Each plant holds a story, a gift, and a purpose. These herbs invite us to listen, to learn, and to grow in rhythm with the earth.

The next herb in our journey is a true healer, known for its sunny disposition and its ability to soothe both body and spirit—**Calendula**.

Why Grow It?

Calendula is the skin whisperer. Its cheerful orange blooms are not only easy to grow, but they also carry potent anti-inflammatory and skin-healing properties. Infused into oils or teas, calendula works wonders for cuts, rashes, and inflammation. Bonus: it attracts pollinators and repels pests in the garden, making it both beautiful and beneficial.

Plant Profile

- **Common Names:** Pot Marigold, Gold Bloom, Mary's Gold
- **Family:** Asteraceae (Daisy family)
- **Parts Used:** Flowers (fresh or dried)
- **Energetics:** Warming, drying
- **Taste:** Slightly bitter, resinous, sweet

Botanical Description

Calendula is a vibrant, sun-loving annual with bright orange or yellow daisy-like flowers.
Its sticky, resin-rich petals are what give it such potent healing power. Native to the Mediterranean, it now thrives in gardens around the world and self-seeds generously.

Grow Tip: Prefers full sun and regular deadheading. Calendula grows easily from seed, making it an ideal addition to any garden.

Medicinal Uses

1. Skin Healing Superstar

Calendula is a topical powerhouse, known for its ability to:

- Speed tissue repair and reduce inflammation
- Soothe cuts, scrapes, burns, eczema, and diaper rashes
- Prevent infection while promoting healing

How to Use: Infuse calendula flowers in oil (like olive or jojoba) and make a balm or salve.

2. Lymphatic and Anti-inflammatory Support

Internally, calendula supports the lymphatic system and can help reduce swollen glands. It's especially helpful for:

- Flu recovery
- Detox protocols
- Acne related to sluggish lymph or poor digestion

3. Digestive and Liver Support

Calendula stimulates liver function and supports gut healing:

- Promotes bile production in the gallbladder
- Soothes inflammation in the gut lining
- Supports detox pathways

How to Use: Drink calendula tea or take a tincture for digestive support.

4. Baby Skincare

Gentle enough for baby care - Use calendula in balms, diaper creams, and rash sprays

How to Use: Infused oil or calendula hydrosol for daily baby skincare.

5. Herbal Bath or Sitz Bath

Calendula is perfect for soothing irritated skin:

- Add to bathwater for full-body relief or sitz baths for postpartum soreness, hemorrhoids, or yeast imbalances.

How to Use: Steep a handful of calendula in hot water and add to bath or compress for sore areas.

6. Soothing Facial Toner or Spray

Calendula tea can be used as a facial toner:

- Reduces inflammation, calms breakouts, and promotes healing.

How to Use: Brew strong calendula tea, cool it, and spritz on skin as a refreshing toner.

7. Infused Honey or Vinegar

Calendula-infused honey or vinegar creates antimicrobial syrups or digestive tonics.

How to Use: Steep dried calendula in raw honey or apple cider vinegar for 1-2 weeks.

8. Natural Dye & Culinary Garnish

Calendula's vibrant petals are a natural dye for Oils, bath salts, soaps, and even food

How to Use: Sprinkle dried petals on breads, soups, or herbal butters for color and cheer.

Traditional & Folk Uses

- Worn as a flower crown for protection and prophetic dreams
- Used in European folk medicine to brighten the spirit and ease grief
- Associated with sun magic, healing, and the Divine Feminine

Magical & Energetic Associations

- Element: Fire & Water
- Planet: Sun
- Chakra: Solar Plexus, Heart

— Used in spells for healing, optimism, protection, and clarity

How to Use Calendula

Infusion (Tea)

- 1–2 tsp dried flowers per cup of water
- Steep 10–15 minutes, covered
- Drink for lymphatic, digestive, or inflammatory support

Tincture

- Fresh or dried flowers in alcohol (1:2 or 1:5)
- Dose: 30–60 drops up to 3x/day

Oil Infusion / Salve

- Infuse dried petals into oil (olive, jojoba, etc.) for 2–6 weeks
- Strain and use as-is or make into balm or salve

Bath or Compress

- Steep calendula tea and pour into bath or soak a cloth to apply to wounds

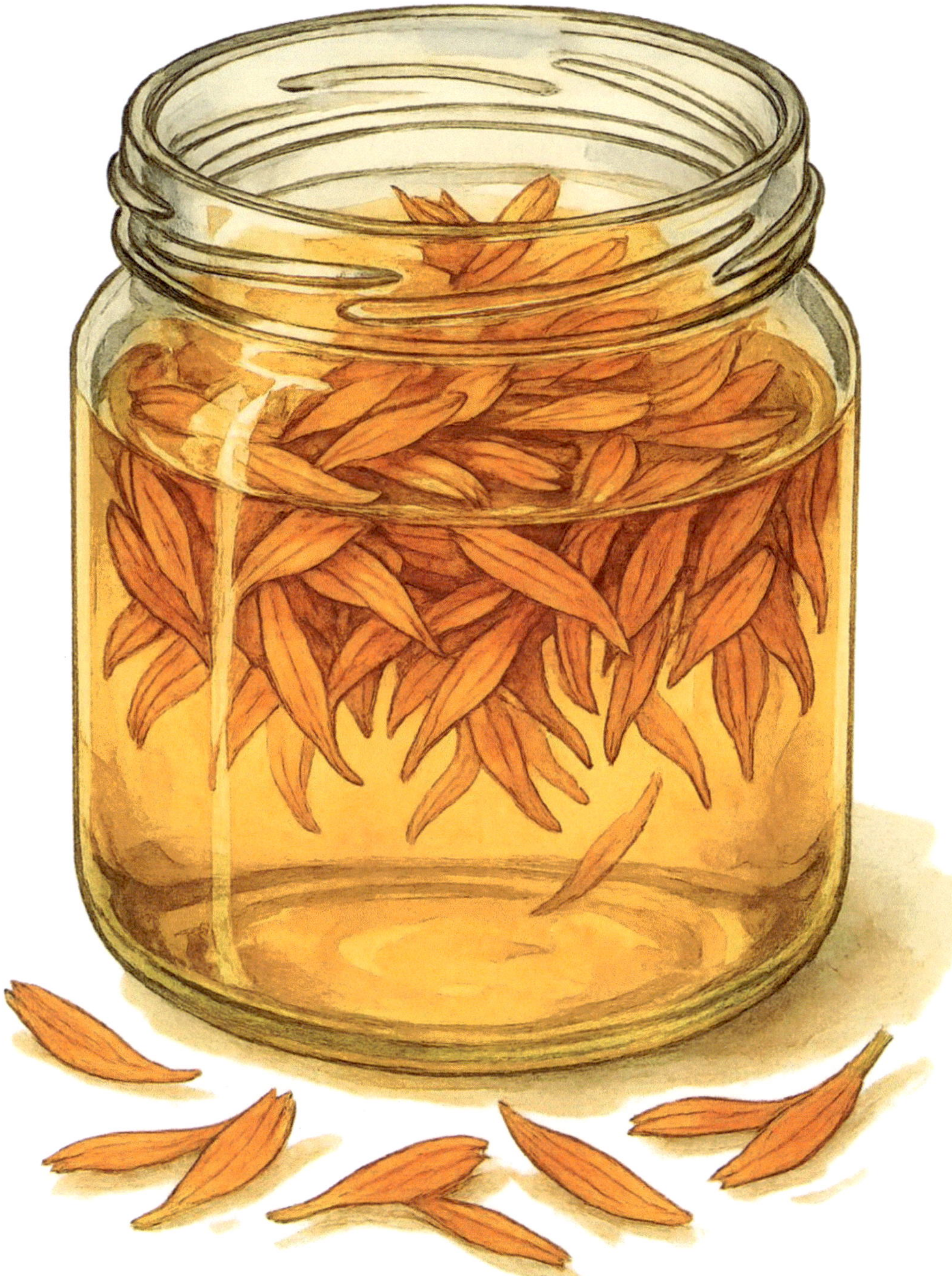

How to Grow Calendula (Pot Marigold)

Calendula (Calendula officinalis) is one of the easiest and most rewarding medicinal herbs to grow. With its cheerful orange blooms and powerful skin-healing properties, calendula thrives in the garden and offers a long blooming season. Whether you're an herbalist, a pollinator enthusiast, or a home apothecary gardener, calendula is an ideal addition.

1. Start from Seed

Calendula is easy to grow from seed, whether you're starting indoors or sowing directly outdoors.

Planting

- **When to Plant:** Calendula prefers cooler temperatures, so plant it in early spring after the danger of frost has passed. You can also sow seeds in late summer for fall blooms. For a continuous display, sow seeds every 2-3 weeks throughout the spring.
- **Starting Indoors:** Sow seeds indoors 4-6 weeks before your last frost date. Plant 1 seed per cell in seed-starting mix, 1/4–1/2 inch deep.
- **Direct Sowing:** Sow seeds directly into your garden bed or containers 1/4 to 1/2 inch deep, spaced 8–12 inches apart.
- **Transplants:** While seeds are recommended, you can also find calendula transplants at garden centers. Plant them after the last frost.

Location & Soil

- **Sunlight:** Calendula thrives in full sun (6–8 hours of direct sunlight) but can tolerate partial shade, especially in hotter climates where afternoon shade may prevent wilting.
- **Soil:** Calendula isn't picky but prefers well-draining, moderately fertile soil with a pH of 6.0–7.0. Amend sandy or clay-like soil with compost for better drainage. Avoid overly rich soil, as too much nitrogen can lead to more foliage and fewer flowers.

Watering

- **Initial Watering:** Water regularly until plants are established.
- **Established Plants:** Calendula is relatively drought-tolerant once established but prefers consistent moisture. Aim for 1 to 1.5 inches of water per week in mid-summer. Avoid overwatering, as soggy soil can lead to root rot.

Care & Maintenance

- **Thinning:** Thin seedlings to 8–12 inches apart to ensure proper airflow and plant development.
- **Deadheading:** Regularly remove spent flowers (deadhead) to encourage continuous blooming. Leave some flowers to go to seed if you want to collect them.

- **Fertilizing:** Calendula isn't a heavy feeder. Apply a balanced, all-purpose fertilizer monthly during the growing season. Use a slow-release granular fertilizer at planting time.
- **Pests & Diseases:** Calendula is generally resilient, but watch out for powdery mildew in humid conditions. Ensure proper spacing and air circulation to prevent this. Aphids can also be an issue—some gardeners use calendula as a trap crop to draw aphids away from other plants.
- **Cold Hardiness:** Calendula can tolerate light frosts and may continue blooming through the first hard freeze.

2. Harvesting

Harvest calendula flower heads when they are fully open. You can use them fresh or dry them for later use in teas, oils, salves, or as a natural dye.

3. Self-Seeding

Calendula is known to self-seed easily. If you leave some flowers to go to seed, new calendula plants may pop up the following year. You can also prevent self-seeding by deadheading all spent flowers.

How to Sprout Calendula Seeds for Planting

You'll need

- Seed-starting tray or small pots
- Seed-starting mix (light, well-draining)
- Calendula seeds
- Spray bottle or gentle watering can
- Warm location or heat mat (optional but helpful)

Steps

1. **Prepare Containers** - Fill containers with moist seed-starting mix. Lightly pat the surface but don't pack it down too tightly.
2. **Sow Seeds** - Plant seeds ¼ inch deep. Calendula seeds are crescent-shaped and don't need light to germinate, so cover them lightly with soil.
3. **Water Gently** - Use a spray bottle or gentle watering can to keep the soil moist without disturbing the seeds.
4. **Maintain Warmth** - Keep seeds in a warm area (65–75°F / 18–24°C) for optimal germination. A heat mat can speed this up.
5. **Keep Moist** - Mist or lightly water daily until you see sprouts.
6. **Provide Light** - Once the seeds sprout, move them to a bright windowsill or under grow lights.
7. **Transplant** - Once seedlings have 2–3 sets of true leaves, harden them off before transplanting them outdoors.

Can You Eat Sprouted Calendula?

Technically yes, but calendula sprouts aren't commonly eaten as microgreens due to their bitter taste and fuzzy texture. The flowers and petals are the more desirable edible parts, commonly used in:

- Herbal teas
- Salves and oils
- Salad garnishes (fresh petals)
- Natural Dyes

Best Use for Sprouted Calendula

Grow them into mature flowering plants and harvest the resin-rich blooms for your herbal remedies.

Calendula Herbal Tea Sipping Chart

Form	Amount per 8oz Water	Steeping Time	Best for
Fresh Petals	1 tablespoon (chopped)	10–15 minutes	Gentle post-harvest sipping, subtle flavor
Dried Petals	1–2 teaspoons	10–15 minutes	Daily skin, gut support, and lymphatic wellness
Strong Infusion	1–2 tablespoons dried	30–60 minutes (covered)	Deep lymphatic, gut, and skin healing
Cold Brew	2 tbsp fresh or 1 tbsp dried	Steep 4–8 hours in cool water	Cooling summer brew, gentle postpartum tonic

Benefits of Calendula Tea

- Soothes gut lining (ulcers, leaky gut, reflux)
- Supports lymphatic flow and clears skin from the inside out
- Eases inflammation and promotes healing
- Provides gentle antimicrobial and antifungal action

Tips

- Always cover while steeping to preserve resins and volatile oils.
- Strain well, as petals can get fluffy when steeped!
- Pairs beautifully with chamomile, marshmallow, or lemon balm.

Calendula's cheerful blooms and healing properties make it a must-have in any herbalist's garden. With its easy-growing nature and powerful medicinal uses, it offers both beauty and utility in your garden and apothecary.

Safety of Calendula by Age Group

Infants (Under 1 Year) — Topical Only

Calendula-infused oils, salves, or bath teas are commonly used for:

- Diaper rash
- Cradle cap
- Eczema

Always patch-test first and use diluted preparations.
Internal use is generally avoided at this age unless directed by a qualified herbalist.

Children (1–12 Years) — Topical + Mild Internal Use

Calendula is great for:

- Skin irritation, minor wounds, scrapes, and bug bites
- Mild teas, honey infusions, or glycerites for Gut inflammation, Lymphatic support during colds or sluggish immunity

Calendula is gentle enough for children, but always ensure proper dosing and avoid heavy medicinal use.

Teens & Adults

Calendula is **very safe** both internally and externally:

- Used in tea, tincture, infused oils, and skin sprays
- Excellent for Digestive inflammation, Menstrual support (especially in combination with other herbs) and Acne, scars, and sunburn recovery.

Caution:

- Do not use internally during pregnancy in large or medicinal doses.
- Mild topical use is generally considered safe during pregnancy.

Elderly

Calendula is **safe and supportive** for older adults:

- Soothing to fragile, thinning skin
- Helpful for circulation, wound care, and digestive inflammation
- Pairs well with comfrey, yarrow, and plantain for enhanced skin healing

When to Use Caution

- **Pregnancy**
  Topical use is okay, but avoid large internal doses as they may stimulate the uterus. Avoid strong teas or tinctures unless supervised by a practitioner.
- **Allergies**
  Rare, but possible for those sensitive to plants in the Asteraceae family (which includes ragweed, chamomile, and others). Always patch-test and monitor for reactions.

CALENDULA NOTES

Personal Experiences

Preparations Tried

Favorite Uses

Blends / Parings

Harvest Notes

Other thoughts

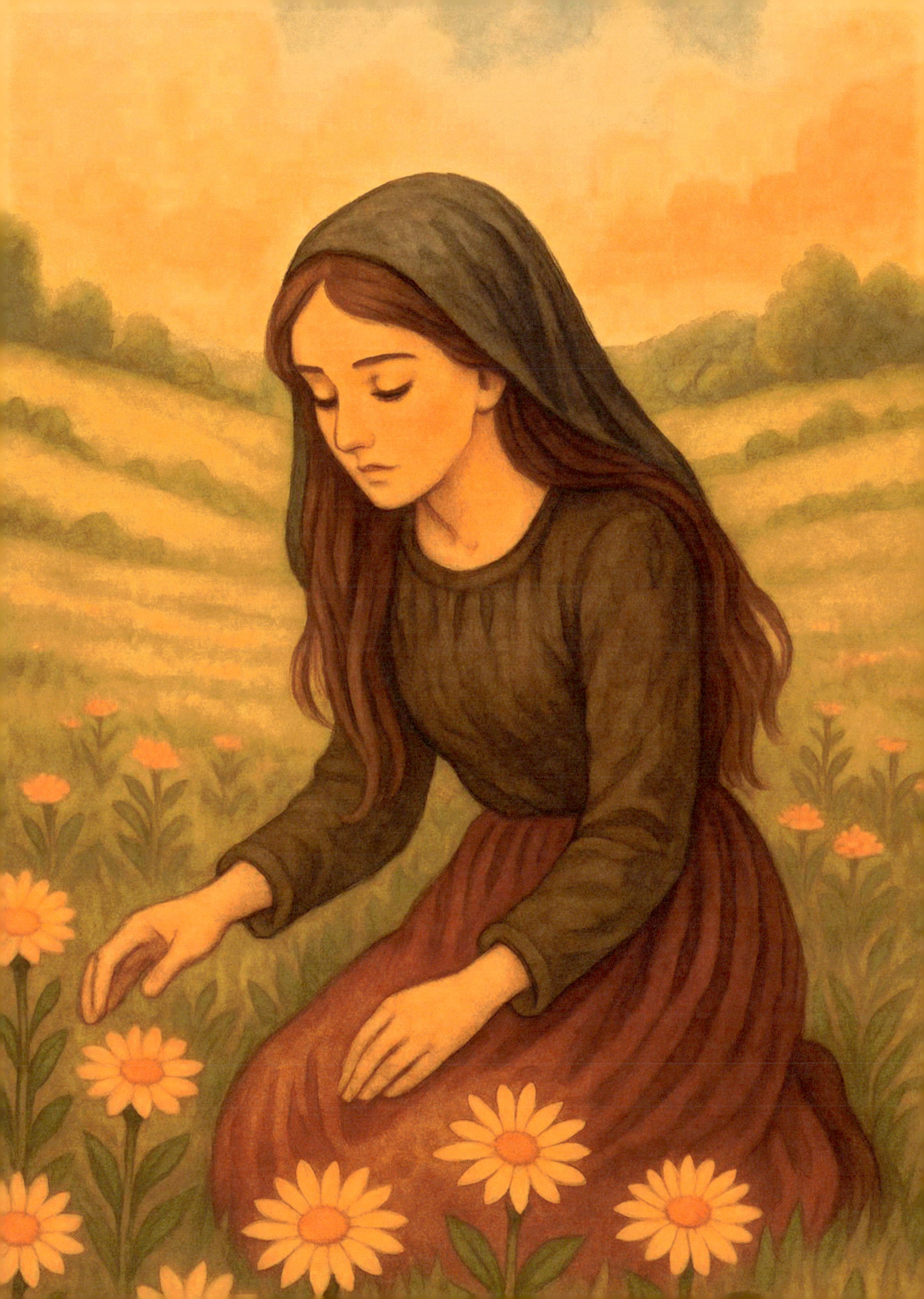

Calendula: The Mourning Maiden and the Sun

Long ago, in a quiet village nestled between the hills, there lived a maiden named Mara. She was known for her laughter and her golden hair, which shimmered like sunlight. She and her beloved, a healer named Lior, were inseparable—gathering herbs, tending to the sick, and singing to the fields as they worked.

But one year, the war came. Lior went to aid the wounded and never returned. Days turned into months, and Mara's laughter faded. Grief filled her heart like heavy rain.

She wandered the fields alone, waiting for a sign, her tears falling into the earth. One morning, at the first light of dawn, Mara collapsed in the meadow where she had once picked wild herbs with Lior. She begged the sun to take her pain and to tell her where love goes when the body is gone.

The sun, moved by her sorrow, wept too. Where their tears mingled, golden flowers bloomed, cupping the sunlight like tiny bowls of hope. These were the first calendulas, born of mourning and love.

The Gift of Calendula

In folk traditions, calendula petals were added to soups and salves for healing. It was tucked into pillows to invite dreams of lost loved ones and scattered across thresholds for protection and blessings.

The name calendula comes from the Latin calendae, meaning "little calendar," for the flower bloomed nearly every day with the sun—reminding us that time, light, and love continue, even after sorrow.

Chamomile

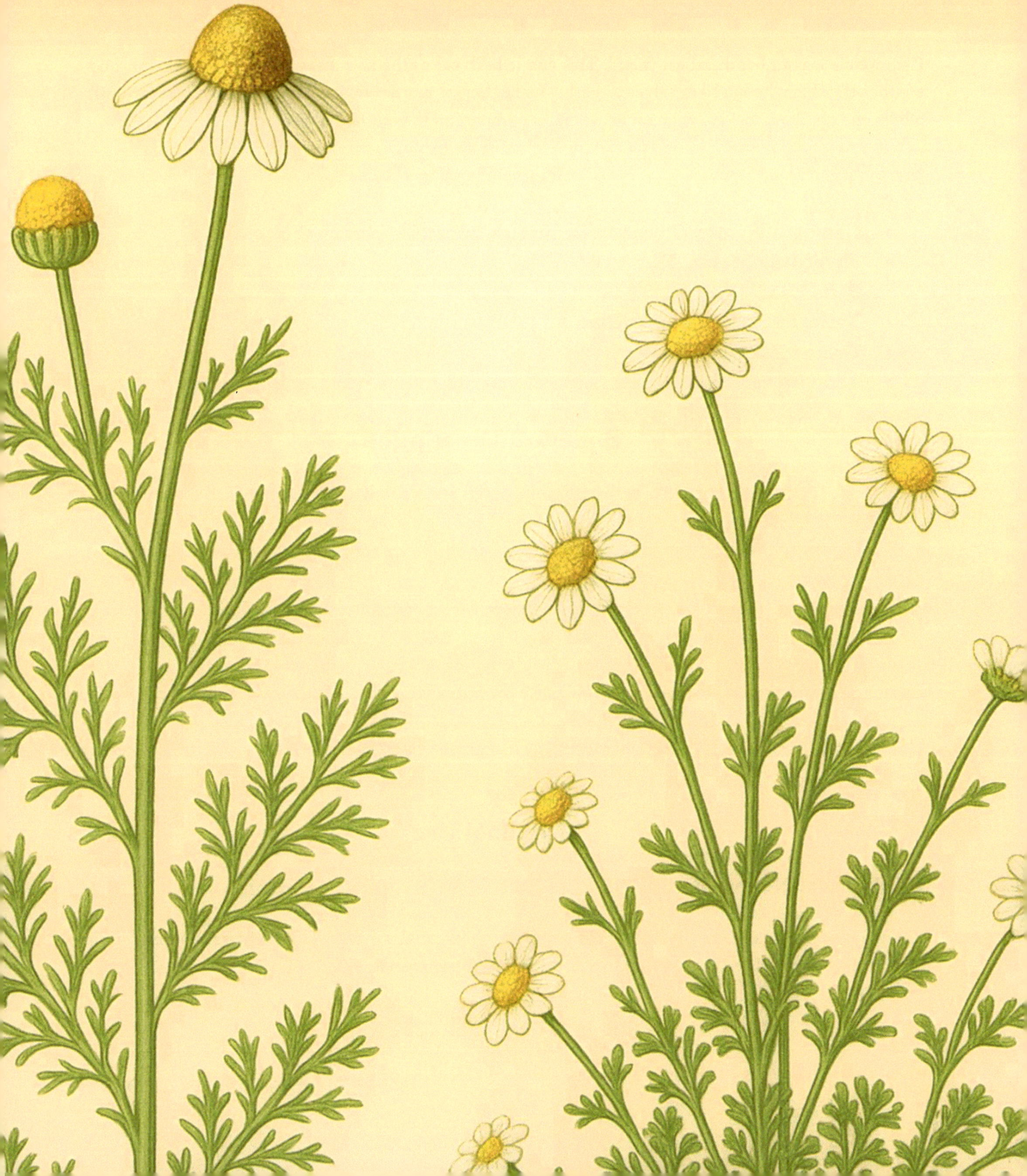

Chamomile (Matricaria chamomilla, Chamaemelum nobile)

Why Grow It?

Chamomile is your bedtime best friend. This gentle herb calms the nervous system, aids digestion, and soothes the skin when used in salves or baths. Its healing properties make it a favorite remedy for both adults and children, making chamomile a perfect companion in your herbal garden.

Plant Profile

- **Common Names:** Ground apple, maythen, manzanilla, physician's plant
- **Family:** Asteraceae (Daisy family)
- **Parts Used:** Flowers
- **Taste:** Sweet, floral, slightly bitter
- **Energetics:** Cooling, drying
- **Actions:** Nervine, carminative, anti-inflammatory, antispasmodic, sedative, vulnerary

Botanical Description

Chamomile is a delicate, daisy-like herb with white petals and a sunny yellow center.

- **German Chamomile** grows upright, reaching 18–24 inches, and is often used in teas and tinctures.
- **Roman Chamomile** is a low-growing perennial ground cover with a similar appearance but a stronger aroma.

Both types share a sweet, apple-like scent—hence the Latin name chamaemelum ("ground apple").

Grow Tip: Chamomile thrives in full sun and well-drained soil. Regular harvesting of flowers ensures the best yield.

Medicinal Uses

1. Calming the Nervous System

Chamomile gently eases anxiety, restlessness, and irritability, making it ideal for bedtime teas and calming both children and adults. It also supports emotional processing and grief.

2. Soothing the Digestive Tract

Safe and effective for babies and elders alike. Chamomile relieves:

- Gas, bloating, indigestion, and nausea
- Colic and IBS
- Tension-related gut discomfort

3. Anti-inflammatory & Skin-Healing

Chamomile works wonders for:

- Eczema, rashes, and minor wounds
- Pink eye (when cooled tea is applied)
- Soothing dry, irritated skin when used in salves, baths, or compresses

4. Sleep Support

- Chamomile's gentle sedative properties help ease into sleep without grogginess.
- Often combined with lemon balm, skullcap, or lavender for dreamy bedtime blends.

Traditional & Folk Uses

- Revered by Egyptians as a sacred herb to Ra, the sun god
- Used in European folklore for luck, protection, and peace
- Believed to banish negativity and promote restful sleep
- Commonly found in charm bags, sleep sachets, and baby baths for peace and protection

Magical & Energetic Associations

- **Element:** Water
- **Planet:** Sun
- **Chakra:** Solar Plexus

— Used for peace, love, purification, restful sleep, and abundance
— Sprinkle around doorways for protection and blessings
— Believed to bring dreams, luck, and calm spirits

How to Use Chamomile

Tea (Infusion)

- 1–2 tsp dried flowers per 8 oz hot water
- Steep, covered, for 5–10 minutes
- Enjoy before bed, after meals, or during times of stress

Tincture

- 1:5 ratio of fresh or dried flowers to alcohol (40–50%)
- Dose: 10–30 drops, up to 3x/day for anxiety, digestion, or sleep

Bath or Compress

- Add strong tea to a bath for stress relief or skin care
- Use cooled tea for eye washes or skin compresses

Oil or Salve

- Infuse dried flowers into oil (e.g., olive or jojoba) for 2–6 weeks
- Strain and use as-is or make into a balm for calming skincare or diaper balm

How to Grow Chamomile

Choose Your Variety

Type	Growth Habit	Best For
German	Tall annual (18–24")	Tea & Tinctures
Roman	Low-growing perennial (4–12")	Groundcover & Gentle Oils

Starting From Seed

German Chamomile

- Start indoors 4–6 weeks before the last frost or sow directly in early spring
- Surface sow—seeds need light to germinate (do not cover heavily)
- Mist lightly and keep the soil moist
- Germinates in 7–14 days

Roman Chamomile

- Can be started from seed or propagated from divisions or nursery plants
- More tolerant of partial shade and poor soil

Growing Conditions

Sun: Full sun is ideal (Roman chamomile tolerates partial shade)
Soil: Well-drained, average to slightly sandy soil—avoid over-fertilizing
Water: Moderate; once established, chamomile is fairly drought-tolerant

Too-rich soil = lots of leafy growth, fewer flowers.

Harvesting

- Harvest when flowers are fully open, preferably in the morning after the dew has dried
- Pick regularly to encourage new blooms
- Dry flowers flat, in a warm, shaded, well-ventilated space
- Store in a sealed jar away from light and heat for best tea and infusion quality

Pollinator & Companion Benefits

- Attracts bees, butterflies, and beneficial insects
- Companion plant to cabbage, onions, and mint
- Gentle enough to grow near sensitive herbs like lavender or lemon balm

Growing Tips

- **German chamomile** self-seeds easily—leave some flowers to go to seed for next year
- **Roman chamomile** can spread as groundcovers—divide every few years to control size

Keep deadheading to extend the bloom season

Suggested Yield

- Expect a small handful of dried flowers per plant per week during peak bloom
- Grow 10+ plants for a year-round supply of tea, salves, and oils

How to Sprout Chamomile Seeds

Chamomile is easy to grow from seed—just provide light, warmth, and patience.

You'll need

- Seed tray or shallow containers
- Seed-starting mix (well-draining, loose)
- Spray bottle or mister
- Chamomile seeds (Matricaria chamomilla or Chamaemelum nobile)
- Plastic dome or clear cover (optional)

Steps:

1. Fill tray with damp seed-starting mix—don't pack it down.
2. Surface sow seeds—chamomile needs light to germinate. Press seeds lightly into the surface.
3. Mist gently—keep the soil moist but not soggy.
4. Cover lightly (optional)—a clear dome helps retain humidity.
5. Place in a warm, sunny area—ideal temperature: 65–70°F (18–21°C).
6. Watch for sprouts—seeds usually germinate in 7–14 days.
7. Thin seedlings once they have 2–3 sets of true leaves—space 4–6 inches apart or transplant into pots or garden.

Bonus Tip:

Sprouting chamomile indoors gives you a head start, especially in cooler climates. Once sprouted, harden off seedlings by gradually exposing them to outdoor conditions before transplanting.

Chamomile's calming and healing properties make it a perfect herb for your garden and your wellness routine. Let it bring peace, healing, and restful sleep into your life.

Can You Eat Chamomile Sprouts?

Technically, yes—chamomile seedlings are not toxic. However, they are:

- Bitter
- Not particularly tender or flavorful
- Not commonly used as microgreens

For the best use, grow chamomile to full bloom and harvest the dried flowers for tea, oil, or skin care.

Chamomile Herbal Tea Sipping Chart

Form	Amount per 8oz Water	Steeping Time	Best for
Fresh Petals	1–2 tablespoons (chopped)	5–7 minutes, covered	Gentle calming tea, skin steams, cooling infusion
Dried Petals	1 tablespoon	7–10 minutes, covered	Deep relaxation, bedtime teas, tincture making
Strong Infusion	1–2 tablespoons dried	30–60 minutes (covered)	Digestive teas, deeper healing
Cold Brew	2 tbsp fresh or 1 tbsp dried	Steep 8–12 hours in refrigerator	Summer sipping, skin soothing toner base

Benefits of Chamomile Tea

- Calms the nervous system
- Supports restful sleep
- Eases digestive woes
- Soothes skin, inside and out
- Relieves PMS & cramps
- Gentle anti-inflammatory properties
- Eases cold & allergy symptoms

Tips: Always cover while steeping to preserve resins and volatile oils for maximum effect.

Safety of Chamomile by Age Group

Infants (Under 1 Year) – Topical Only

Use with caution and only externally or in very dilute form.

- **Uses:** Warm chamomile tea added to bathwater; a few drops of diluted tea on gums for teething
- **Avoid:** Internal use for infants under 6 months due to immature digestion and potential contamination risks
- **Caution:** Chamomile belongs to the Asteraceae family (which includes ragweed). Test a small patch first, especially for infants or individuals with known seasonal allergies.

Toddlers (1–3 Years) – Safe in Small, Diluted Amounts

- **Uses:** Weak tea for colic, restlessness, or teething pain
- **Dosage:** 1–2 oz of weak tea, once per day as needed
- **Form:** Use tea, not essential oils (EOs are too concentrated for this age group)

Children (4–12 Years) – Very Safe in Tea Form

- **Uses:** Anxiety, upset stomach, restlessness, bedtime support
- **Dosage:** 4–6 oz tea, up to 2x daily
- **Optional:** Combine with lemon balm or spearmint for a tasty kids' blend

Teens & Adults (13+)

Safe in all common forms: tea, tincture, capsules, compresses, and baths

- **Uses:** Tea, tincture, sleep support, digestive aid
- **Dosage:** Standard 8 oz tea, up to 3x daily
- **Note:** Watch for increased sedation if combined with other calming herbs or medications

Older Adults (65+) – Gentle and Supportive

- **Uses:** Digestive aid, sleep tea, anti-inflammatory compresses
- **Caution:** May increase drowsiness or interact mildly with sedative medications
- **Form:** Tea is safest; tincture well-tolerated at low doses

Chamomile Allergy Warning

Chamomile is a member of the Asteraceae family, which includes ragweed, daisies, and marigolds. Those with ragweed allergies may react to chamomile. Always patch-test or try a very small amount before using regularly, especially with infants or those with known seasonal allergies.

CHAMOMILE NOTES

Personal Experiences

Preparations Tried

Favorite Uses

Blends / Parings

Harvest Notes

Other thoughts

Chamomile: The Flower That Waited

In a sleepy village where winters were long and harsh, there lived a small, sickly girl named Anya. Often too weak to play, she would watch from her window as others danced in the meadows. Her mother, a weaver of wool and stories, tried every herb and poultice to bring her strength, but Anya remained pale and tired.

One night, the mother dreamed of a golden field under a moonlit sky. In the middle of the field stood a small white flower with a yellow heart, glowing softly like a lantern. A voice whispered: "I grow where others fail. I wait where others wilt. I am small, but I carry the power of the sun."

When the mother awoke, she searched the woods and riverbanks until she found the same delicate flower. It was blooming cheerfully among stones where nothing else dared grow.

She brewed the blossoms into a gentle tea and gave it to Anya. That night, the girl slept peacefully for the first time in many weeks. Each day, the tea brought calm, dreams, and a touch more color to her cheeks. In time, Anya returned to the fields with the others, laughter trailing behind her like wind in tall grass.

Chamomile's Gifts

Chamomile reminds us that true strength doesn't shout. It whispers softly through rest, patience, and healing.

Peppermint

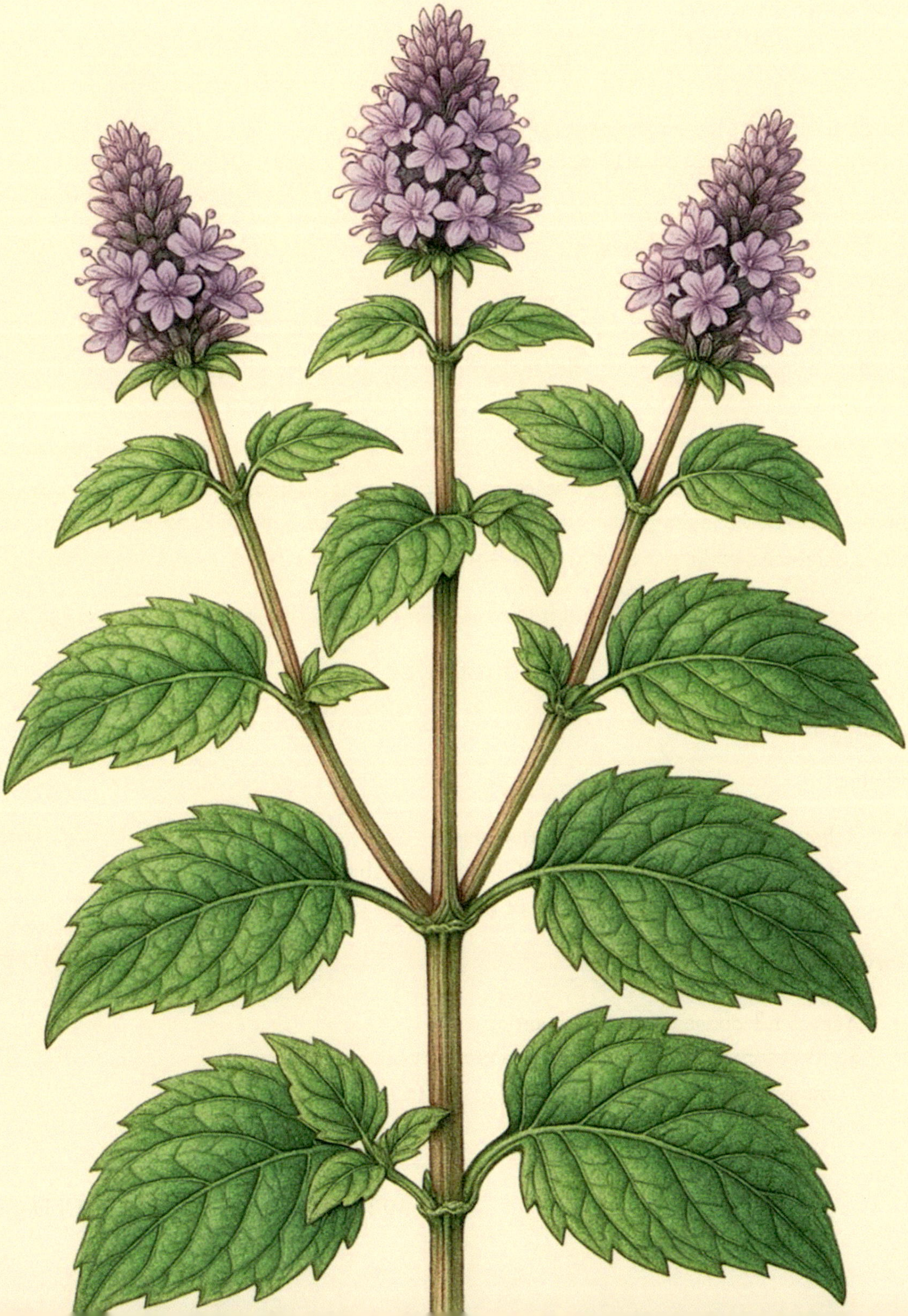

Peppermint
(Mentha x piperita)

Why Grow It?

Peppermint is the digestive champion of the garden. It's a go-to remedy for headaches, nausea, and bloating. Its cooling properties also make it excellent in salves or foot soaks. The scent alone can lift fatigue, clear your mind, and revive the senses.

Plant Profile

- Botanical Name: Mentha × piperita
- Common Names: Peppermint, Brandy Mint
- Family: Lamiaceae (Mint family)
- Parts Used: Leaves, flowering tops
- Taste: Cool, pungent, slightly sweet
- Energetics: Cooling, drying
- Actions: Carminative, antispasmodic, analgesic, antimicrobial, nervine, decongestant

Botanical Description

Peppermint is a hybrid of spearmint (Mentha spicata) and watermint (Mentha aquatica). It has square stems, dark green pointed leaves with a sharp menthol scent, and purple-tinged flowers. Peppermint spreads rapidly via underground rhizomes, making it easy to grow—sometimes too easy!

Grow Tip: Peppermint grows vigorously. Plant it in containers to control its spread.

Medicinal Uses

1. Digestive Support

Peppermint helps:

- Relieve gas, bloating, cramping, and nausea
- Calm irritable bowel syndrome (IBS) and stomach tension
- Commonly used in post-meal tea or tinctures for digestive support

2. Respiratory Relief

- Acts as a decongestant and expectorant
- Soothes sore throats and eases sinus pressure
- Commonly used in steam blends, salves, or teas for respiratory health

3. Headache & Mental Fatigue

- Peppermint's cooling properties ease tension headache
- Cooled tea compresses or diluted essential oil can help relieve pain
- Mentally stimulating, peppermint clears brain fog and boosts focus

4. Nervous System Support

- Gently uplifting without sedation
- Soothes anxiety and overstimulation when paired with chamomile or lemon balm

Traditional & Folk Uses

- Used since ancient Egypt for indigestion and breath freshening
- Worn or carried to ward off evil or illness
- Believed to promote healing, energetic refreshment, and clarity
- Associated with clarity, movement, and transformation

Magical & Energetic Associations

- **Element:** Air
- **Planet:** Mercury
- **Chakra:** Throat & Third Eye

— Used for clarity, purification, protection, mental sharpness, and energy clearing
— Excellent for cleansing baths, spell work, or altar offerings
— Burned in rituals for purification and renewal
— Used in charm bags to break hexes, bring luck, or attract prosperity
— Slipped into shoes or bathwater to refresh the body and awaken the soul

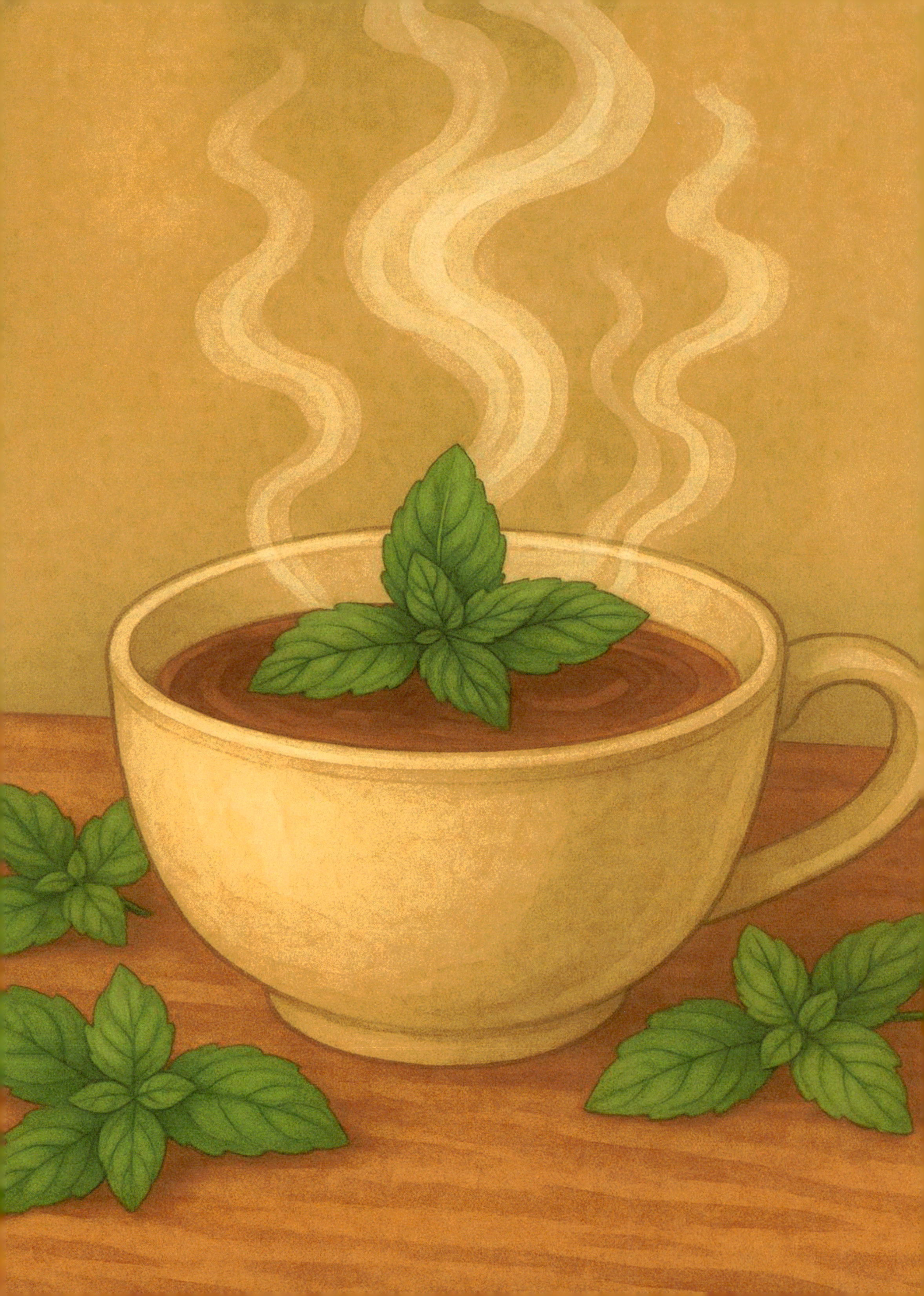

How to Use Peppermint

Infusion (Tea)

- 1 tsp dried or 1 tbsp fresh per 8 oz water
- Steep covered for 10–15 minutes
- Drink hot or cold for digestion, clarity, or cold support

Tincture

- 1:5 in 40–50% alcohol
- Dose: 10–30 drops as needed

Steam / Compress

- Add to boiling water and inhale steam for sinus relief
- Use cooled tea compresses on head or belly

Infused Oil / Salve

- Combine with rosemary or eucalyptus for congestion, sore muscles, or tension

How to Grow Peppermint

Growing from Cuttings (Best Method)

Peppermint is most often propagated from cuttings or root divisions, as it is a sterile hybrid and rarely produces viable seeds.

Steps to Root a Cutting

1. Take a 4–6 inch stem cutting from a healthy plant
2. Remove bottom leaves and place in water or moist potting soil
3. Roots will develop in 7–14 days
4. Transplant into a garden or container once roots are well established

Growing from Seed

Most peppermint seeds sold are a mix of spearmint and other mints, but if you have labeled peppermint seeds:

- Sow indoors 6–8 weeks before the last frost
- Press seeds into the soil surface (needs light to germinate)
- Keep moist, germination takes 10–16 days
- Thin seedlings to strongest plants and transplant when 2–3" tall

Growing Conditions

- Sun: Full sun is ideal (Roman peppermint tolerates part shade)
- Soil: Well-drained, slightly sandy soil—avoid over-fertilizing
- Water: Moderate; once established, peppermint is fairly drought-tolerant
  Too-rich soil = excessive leafy growth, fewer flowers.

Harvesting

- Harvest peppermint when flowers are just beginning to open
- Pick regularly to encourage new blooms
- Dry flowers flat, in a warm, shaded, well-ventilated space
- Store in a sealed jar away from light and heat for best quality

Pollinator & Companion Benefits

- Attracts bees, butterflies, and beneficial insects
- Companion plant to cabbage, onions, and mint
- Gentle enough to grow near sensitive herbs like lavender or lemon balm

Growing Tips

- German peppermint self-seeds easily—let some flowers go to seed for next year
- Roman peppermint can spread as groundcovers—divide every few years to control size
- Keep deadheading to extend the bloom season

Suggested Yield

- Expect a small handful of dried flowers per plant per week during peak bloom
- Grow 10+ plants if you want to make salves, oils, and tea year-round

How to Sprout Peppermint Seeds

Peppermint is easy to grow from seed. Just provide light, warmth, and patience.

You'll need:

- Seed tray or shallow containers
- Seed-starting mix (well-draining, loose)
- Spray bottle or mister
- Peppermint seeds (Mentha × piperita)
- Plastic dome or clear cover (optional)

Steps:

1. Fill tray with damp seed-starting mix—don't pack it down.
2. Surface sow seeds—press lightly into the soil.
3. Mist gently—keep the soil moist but not soggy.
4. Cover lightly (optional)—a clear dome helps retain humidity.
5. Place in a warm, sunny area (65–70°F / 18–21°C).
6. Watch for sprouts—seeds usually germinate in 7–14 days.
7. Thin seedlings once they have 2–3 sets of true leaves—space 4–6 inches apart or transplant into pots or the garden.

Bonus Tip: Sprouting peppermint indoors gives you a head start, especially in cooler climates. Once sprouted, harden off seedlings by gradually exposing them to outdoor conditions before transplanting.

Sprouting Peppermint from Seed **(Not Ideal)**

Here's the catch:

- Seeds labeled "peppermint" are often not true peppermint but a mix of spearmint and other mints.
- Even if you find true peppermint seeds, germination rates can be low, and the plants may not resemble the parent plant.

If you're still starting from seed:

- **Surface sow**—press seeds into moist soil but don't cover them (they need light).
- Keep warm and mist regularly.
- Germination can take 10–16+ days.
- **Thin** to the strongest seedlings and transplant when they're about 2–3 inches tall.

Can You Eat Peppermint Sprouts?

Technically, yes, but:

- They grow very slowly.
- They're not commonly eaten as microgreens.
- Peppermint is best used when fully mature, as this is when its essential oil content is the highest.

Summary: Best Way to "Sprout" Peppermint

Method	**Reliable?**	**Notes**
Cuttings	Yes	Fast, easy, identical to parent
Division	Yes	Works well for mature plants
Seeds	Not Ideal	Often mislabeled, variable traits

Peppermint Herbal Tea Sipping Chart

Form	Amount per 8oz Water	Steeping Time	Best For
Fresh Petals	1 tsp – 1 Tbsp (chopped)	5–10 minutes	Bold, concentrated flavor
Dried Petals	1 Tbsp–1/4 cup loosely packed	5–10 minutes	Light, green, aromatic flavor
Strong Infusion	2x regular amount	15–20 minutes (covered)	Robust, medicinal flavor
Cold Brew	1 Tbsp–1/4 cup loosely packed	Steep 4–12 hours in cool water	Refreshing summer sipping, hydration

Benefits of Peppermint Tea

- Soothes digestion
- Relieves headaches
- Freshens breath
- Reduces nausea
- Clears nasal congestion
- Eases menstrual cramps
- Enhances focus and alertness
- Supports liver and gallbladder health
- Caffeine-free comfort
- Anti-spasmodic properties

Safety of Peppermint by Age Group

Infants (Under 3 Years Old) – Topical Only

Peppermint is not recommended for infants as it may irritate the stomach. Additionally, menthol can slow breathing and irritate sensitive systems.

Children (4–7 Years) – Topical + Mild Internal Use

- Peppermint tea is generally safe in small, diluted amounts (about 1–2 ounces at a time).
- Topical use of diluted peppermint oil (1–2%) may be acceptable, but a patch test is essential.

Children (8–12 Years) – Topical + Mild Internal Use

- Safe to enjoy peppermint tea in moderate amounts (4–6 ounces).
- May benefit from diluted topical applications (1–3%) for sore muscles or mild headaches.

Teens, Adults, and Elderly (13+)

- Peppermint is typically safe in all common forms, including tea and diluted oil.
- Those with acid reflux or GERD may want to limit peppermint use, as it can relax the esophageal sphincter and worsen symptoms.

When to Use Caution

- **During Pregnancy or Nursing:** Peppermint tea may be safe in light amounts, but opinions vary. It's best to consult with a healthcare provider.

Topical Use: Peppermint oil should be spot-tested and avoided on the abdomen during pregnancy.

PEPPERMINT NOTES

Personal Experiences

Preparations Tried

Favorite Uses

Blends / Parings

Harvest Notes

Other thoughts

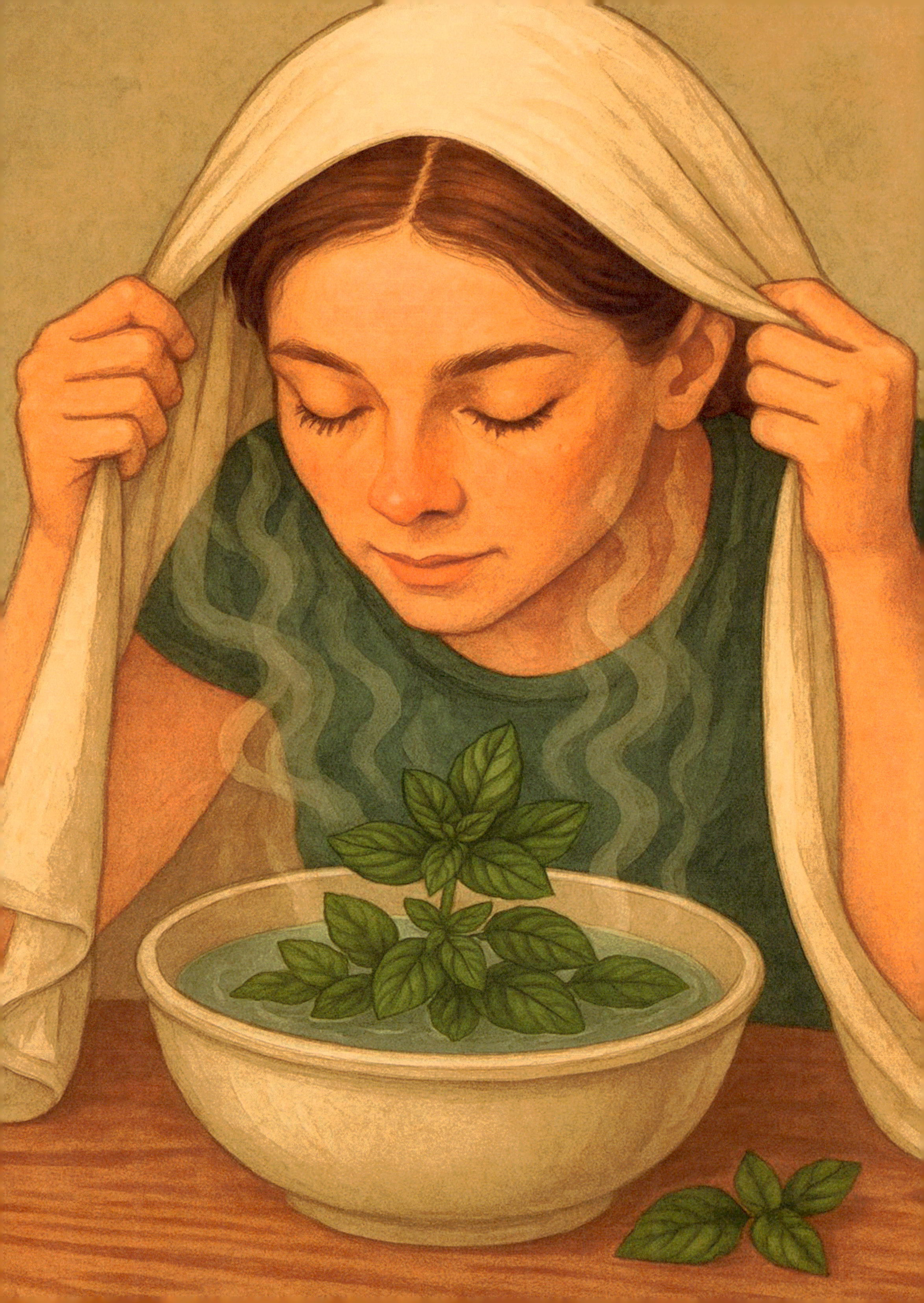

Peppermint: The Nymph of Sweet Waters

In the time of gods and green hills, there lived a beautiful water nymph named Minthe. She danced in the cool streams, and with her laughter, she scented the air. Her presence was so refreshing that wild animals would stop to rest near her waters, and travelers swore their fatigue lifted after a sip from her spring.

But Minthe caught the attention of Hades, the god of the underworld. He was drawn to her cool beauty and wild spirit. In some versions of the folk tale, Hades courted her; in others, he tried to claim her. Regardless, Persephone, his queen, saw the encounter and grew jealous.

With a wave of her hand, Persephone cast a spell on Minthe, transforming her into a low-growing, humble herb. No longer could Minthe dance or shimmer. She would live forever underfoot.

Yet the gods underestimated Minthe's spirit.

Where she had been cast down, the ground grew lush and green, and the air filled with a bright, clean scent. Anyone who stepped near would feel refreshed, uplifted, and alert.

Minthe, now Peppermint, had not been silenced. She had become something new—a healer, a purifier, and a breath of clarity.

Peppermint Whispers

When life casts you low, root deep, rise fragrant, and bring sweetness wherever your feet now tread.

HOLY BASIL

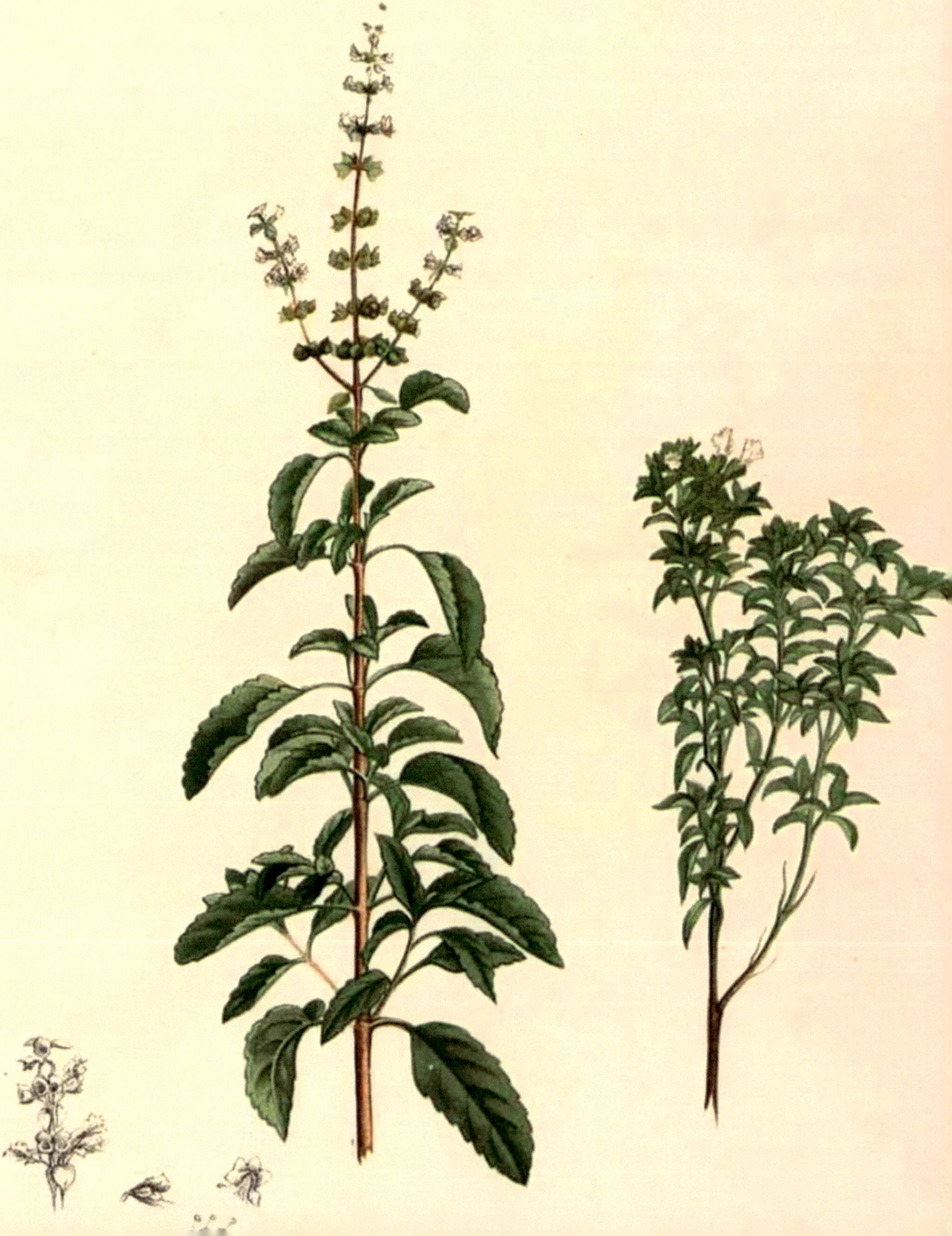

Holy Basil (Ocimum sanctum/Ocimum tenuiflorum)

Why Grow It?

Tulsi is sacred for a reason. Revered in Ayurveda, this adaptogen helps the body cope with stress, enhances mental clarity, and supports immunity. The tea alone is a daily ritual in many homes, offering peace, protection, and balance.

Plant Profile

- **Botanical Name:** Ocimum sanctum / Ocimum tenuiflorum
- **Common Names:** Tulsi, Sacred Basil, Queen of Herbs
- **Family:** Lamiaceae (Mint family)
- **Parts Used:** Leaves, flowers, stems (fresh or dried)
- **Taste:** Spicy, slightly sweet, clove-like
- **Energetics:** Warming, drying
- **Actions:** Adaptogen, nervine, carminative, immunomodulator, antimicrobial, uplifting

Botanical Description

Holy Basil is a fragrant, shrubby annual or short-lived perennial with green or purple-tinged leaves and purple flowers. Native to India and Southeast Asia, it has been revered for over 3,000 years in Ayurvedic medicine and Hindu tradition as a sacred plant of protection, devotion, and vitality.

Grow Tip: Tulsi loves heat and sunlight. Pinch off flowers to encourage lush, leafy growth.

Medicinal Uses

1. Stress & Emotional Resilience

- A powerful adaptogen that helps the body adapt to physical, emotional, and environmental stress
- Lifts the mood, balances cortisol, and promotes a clear, calm mind
- Especially helpful for burnout, anxiety, or spiritual fatigue

2. Immune Support

- Modulates immune function — neither overstimulating nor suppressing
- Used preventively and during colds, flus, or respiratory infections

3. Respiratory & Anti-inflammatory

- Eases cough, congestion, and asthma-like symptoms
- Naturally antiviral, antibacterial, and anti-inflammatory

Magical & Energetic Associations

- **Element:** Fire & Spirit
- **Planet:** Mercury & Jupiter
- **Chakras:** Heart, Crown

— Used for cleansing, spiritual protection, devotion, clarity, and joy
— Said to open the heart, purify the aura, and connect to the divine
— Known to protect against evil, illness, and despair—Tulsi is as much a guardian as she is a healer.

Traditional Uses

- Tulsi is one of the most sacred herbs in Ayurveda and Hinduism
- Grown in household altars to protect the home and purify energy
- Offered to deities and used in spiritual bathing, ceremonies, and healing

How to Use Holy Basil

Infusion (Tea)

- 1 tbsp dried herb per 8–10 oz hot water
- Steep covered for 10–15 minutes
- Drink daily for mood, immunity, and nervous system support

Tincture

- Fresh or dried in alcohol (1:2 to 1:5 ratio)
- Dose: 30–60 drops, up to 3x/day

Infused Honey / Oxymel

- Combine with ginger or lemon balm for an uplifting herbal elixir

Fresh Use

- Can be chewed fresh or made into a cooling summer drink (like Tulsi lemonade!)

How to Grow Holy Basil (Tulsi)

Tulsi thrives in warm, sunny environments, and it's easy to grow with the right care—whether in containers, garden beds, or a sunny windowsill.

Start from Seed

- **Indoors:** Start 6–8 weeks before your last frost date
- **Outdoors:** After the danger of frost has passed

Steps:

1. Fill seed trays with moist, well-draining seed-starting mix.
2. Surface sow—press seeds lightly into the soil (they need light to germinate).
3. Mist gently and keep the soil moist.
4. Keep in a warm spot (70–80°F). Heat mats help speed up germination.
5. Germination in 7–14 days.

How to Sprout Holy Basil (Tulsi) from Seed

Holy basil is easy to start from seed indoors or directly in the garden (in warm climates).

You'll need

- Holy basil seeds
- Seed-starting mix (light, well-draining)
- Seed trays or pots
- Spray bottle or gentle watering can
- Heat mat or sunny window

Step-by-Step Instructions

1. Start indoors 6–8 weeks before the last frost date (or direct sow outdoors after frost if soil is warm).
2. Fill trays with moist seed-starting mix (don't overpack it).
3. Surface sow the seeds—press gently into the soil.
4. Mist gently to keep the surface moist (not soggy).
5. Keep warm and bright (ideal temperature: 70–80°F).
6. Germination usually takes 7–14 days, sometimes longer in cooler temperatures.
7. Thin seedlings once they have 2–3 sets of true leaves.

After Sprouting:

- Transplant outdoors after danger of frost has passed.
- Space plants 12–18 inches apart in full sun.
- Water when the top inch of soil is dry.
- Harvest regularly to encourage bushy growth.

Can You Eat Tulsi Sprouts?

Technically, yes, but:

- The flavor is strong and spicy, like clove and cinnamon.
- Tulsi is much more valuable as a mature herb for teas, oils, and tinctures.

Growing Tips for Success

Tip	Why It Helps
Don't cover the seeds	They need light to germinate
Use bottom heat	Encourages faster and more even sprouting
Water lightly	Prevents mold and rot
Be patient	Tulsi germinates slower than sweet basil

Holy Basil (Tulsi) Tea Sipping Chart

Form	Amount per 8oz Water	Steeping Time	Best for
Fresh Petals	1 Tbsp – ¼ cup loosely packed	7–10 minutes	Warm, slightly sweet, clove-like flavor
Dried Petals	1 tsp – 1 Tbsp (chopped)	7–10 minutes	Earthy, medicinal, deeper tone
Strong Infusion	1–2 tablespoons dried	30–60 minutes (covered)	Earthy, medicinal, deeper tone
Cold Brew	1 tbsp dried	Steep 6–12 hours in cool water	Cooling summer brew, gentle daily sipping

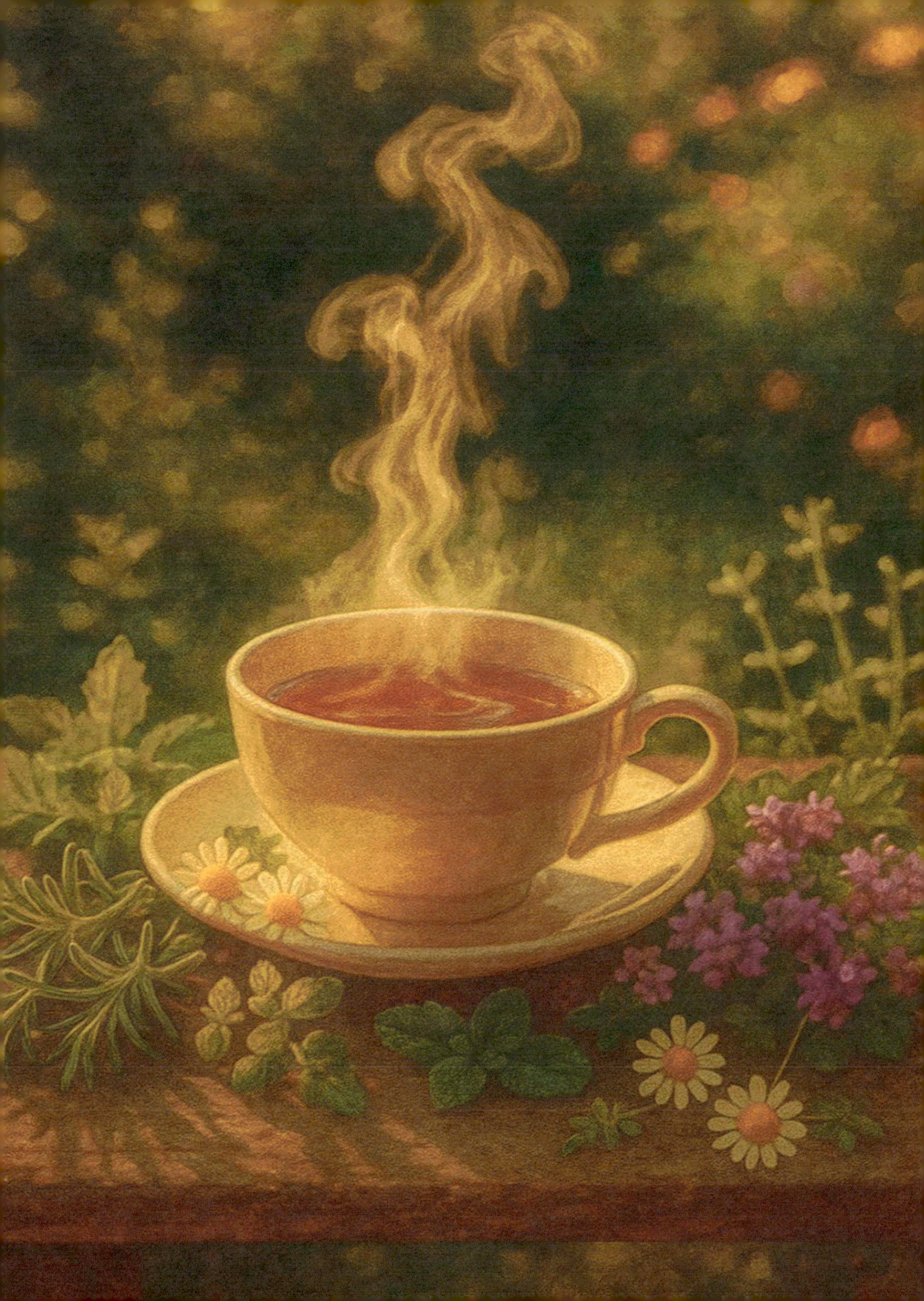

Benefits of Tulsi Tea

- Stress relief & Adaptogenic support
- Immune support
- Balances blood sugar & metabolism
- Supports respiratory health
- Heart & circulatory support
- Cognitive clarity & mood boosting
- Anti-inflammatory & pain relief
- Gut & digestive tonic
- Antioxidant-rich cellular protection
- Gentle detoxifier

Safety of Tulsi by Age Group

Infants (0–12 Months)

- Not recommended.
- Tulsi is too stimulating and potentially drying for infants. While it has antimicrobial and immune-boosting benefits, their systems are too delicate for herbal teas or tinctures. Avoid all forms of internal use unless guided by a pediatric herbalist.

Toddlers (1–3 Years)

Use with caution and only in very mild forms.

- Small sips of very weak Tulsi tea (1 leaf or a pinch of dried herb steeped briefly) may be used occasionally for immune support or mild colds, but it should not be part of a toddler's daily routine.
- Topical preparations like Tulsi-infused oil may be used externally in diluted form for chest rubs or calming massage. Avoid essential oils entirely.

Children (4–7 Years)

Light use is generally safe.

- Children in this age group can enjoy mild Tulsi tea, especially during colds, overstimulation, or seasonal transitions. Limit to 2–4 oz at a time, steeped lightly.
- Tulsi glycerites (alcohol-free tinctures) may also be used in small doses.
- Topical use is generally well-tolerated, but essential oil should still be avoided due to its potency.

Older Children (8–12 Years)

- Safe in moderate amounts.
- Children 8 and up can safely enjoy 1 cup of Tulsi tea daily, particularly during times of stress, study, or immune challenge.
- Tulsi's Adaptogenic nature supports emotional resilience and focus.
- Tinctures and salves are appropriate when diluted. Light diffusion of Tulsi essential oil may be introduced under supervision.

Teens (13–18 Years)

Well-tolerated and beneficial.

- Tulsi is a wonderful ally for teens dealing with emotional stress, academic pressure, or shifting immune needs.
- 1–2 cups of tea per day is safe, or 10–20 drops of tincture as needed.
- Topical preparations are helpful for skin issues and stress tension. Essential oil should be used cautiously—always diluted and never ingested.

Adults (19–64 Years)

Safe and supportive for daily use.

- Tulsi is a cornerstone of adult herbal wellness. It can be consumed daily as tea, tincture, or capsule, supporting the nervous system, hormones, metabolism, and immunity.
- Most adults tolerate 1–3 cups of tea per day or 30–60 drops of tincture.
- It pairs well with other adaptogens and can be used topically for inflammation or added to skincare.
- Caution: Those with low blood sugar, hypothyroidism, or on medications should consult a practitioner, as Tulsi may influence insulin sensitivity and hormone levels.

Elderly Adults (65+)

Gentle and supportive with minor precautions.

- Tulsi can be very beneficial in older adults for improving cognitive clarity, supporting heart health, and reducing inflammation.
- Start with small servings of tea (4–6 oz) and monitor how the body responds. Tulsi is also useful for uplifting mood and supporting detox pathways that may slow with age.

Pregnancy & Nursing

Use with caution and guidance.

- Tulsi has a long history in traditional systems, but its use in pregnancy is debated.
- Some sources advise avoiding it due to possible uterine-stimulating effects and its influence on hormone balance.
- Others allow occasional light tea under professional supervision.
- Nursing parents may find Tulsi helpful for stress and immune support, but moderation is key.

BASIL NOTES

Personal Experiences

Preparations Tried

Favorite Uses

Blends / Parings

Harvest Notes

Other thoughts

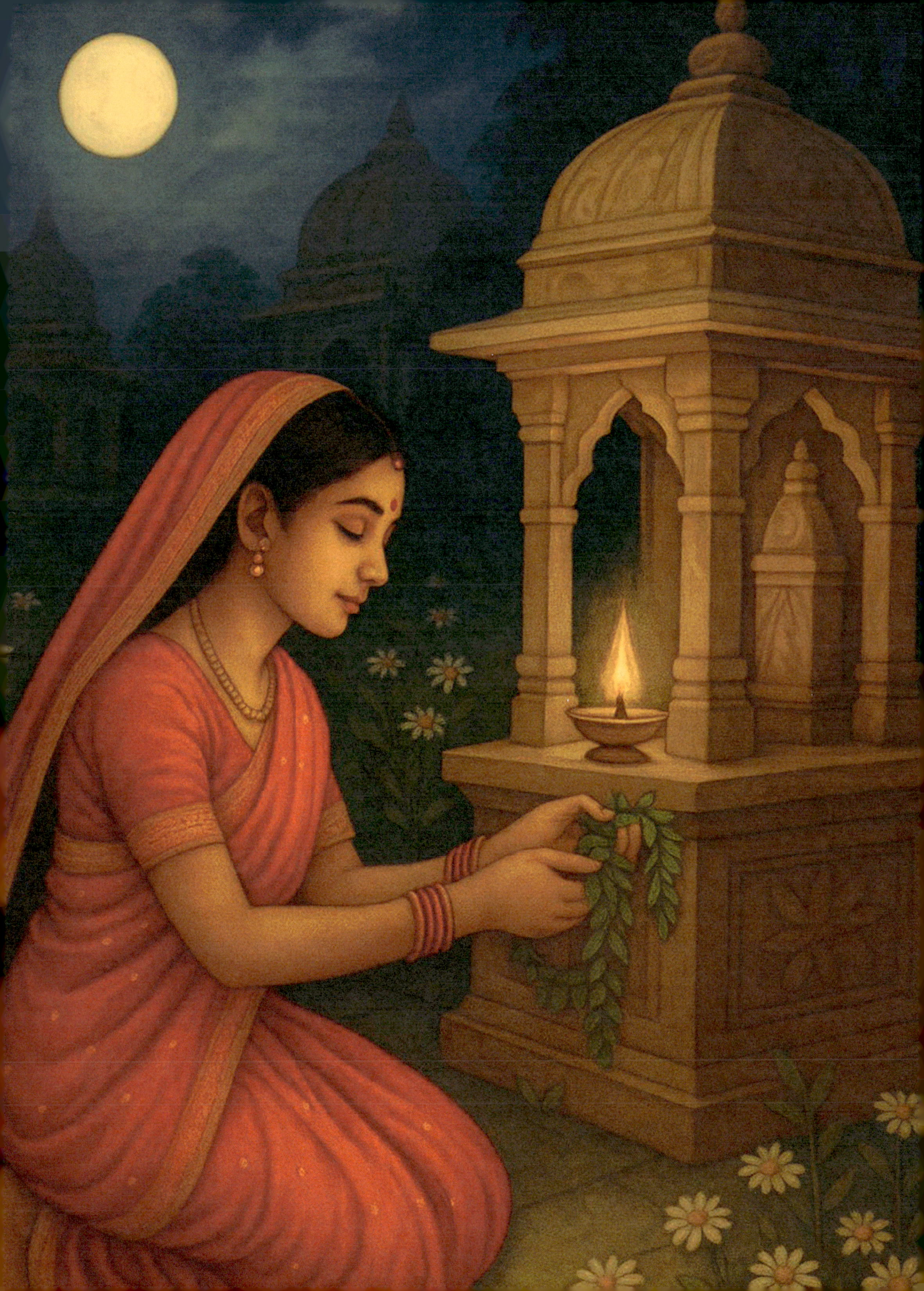

The Tale of Tulsi: The Sacred Bride of Vishnu

Long ago, in the lands of India, there lived a devoted woman named Vrinda. She was the wife of the powerful demon king Jalandhar. Unlike him, Vrinda was pure of heart and utterly devoted to the god Vishnu, the preserver of the universe.

Because of her unwavering virtue and spiritual power, Vrinda's prayers protected her husband from harm, even in battle against the gods. No weapon could touch him as long as her faith remained unshaken.

Desperate to restore balance and defeat the tyrant king, Vishnu took on a human form and appeared before Vrinda. Through divine illusion, he gently broke her faith by disguising himself as her husband. The spell was brief, but it was enough. The moment her purity was broken, Jalandhar lost his divine protection and was defeated in battle.

When Vrinda discovered the deception, her heart shattered. Though she revered Vishnu, she cursed him for the pain and betrayal. Then, overcome by sorrow, she cast herself into the fire.

But Vishnu, full of compassion and remorse, honored her devotion by transforming her soul into a sacred plant: Tulsi—the holiest of herbs.

Tulsi Reminds Us

True devotion has power beyond death. Even heartbreak can become sacred when love is offered with a pure heart.

YARROW

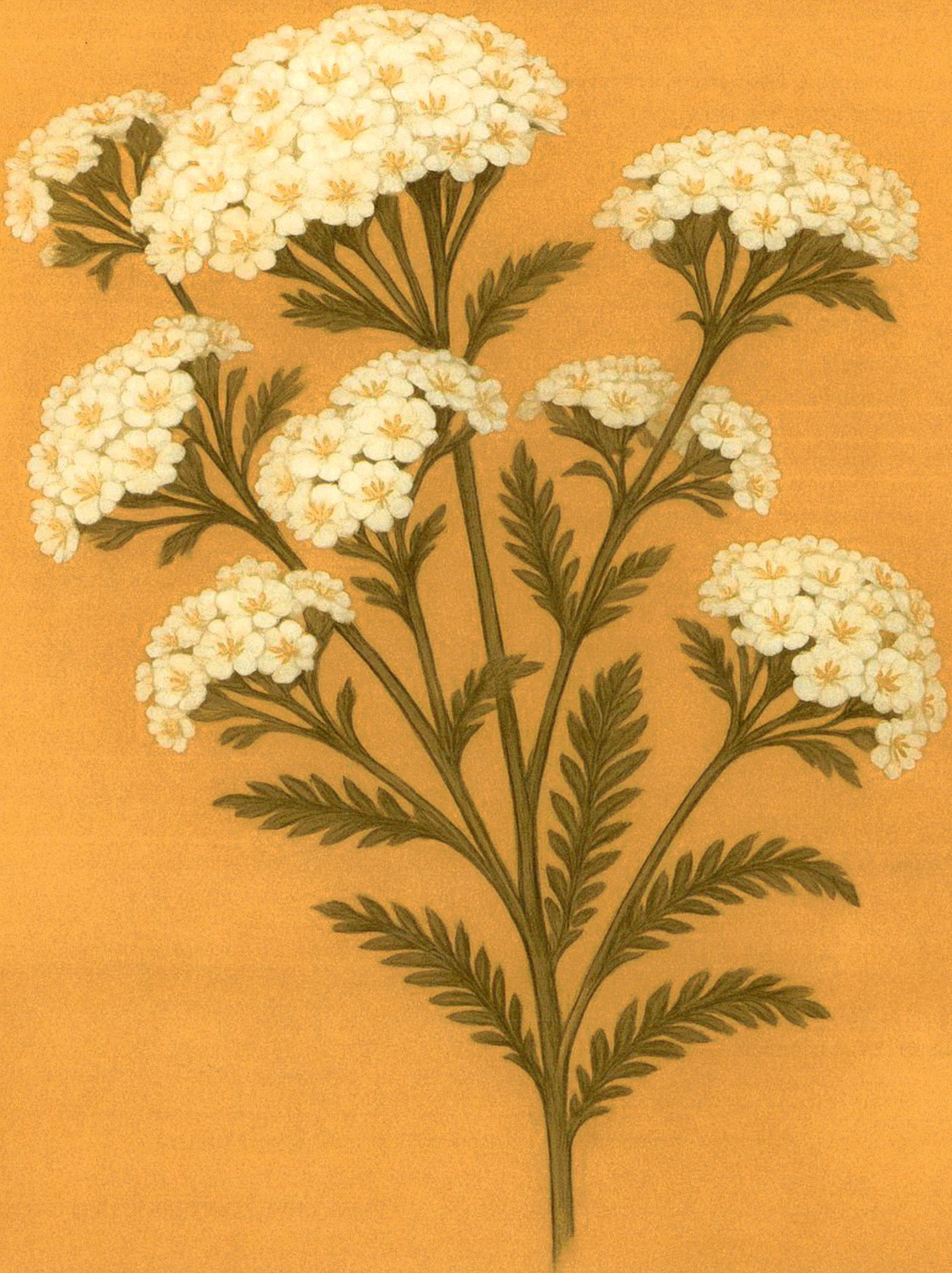

Yarrow
(Achillea millefolium)

Why Grow It?

Yarrow is the first-aid hero of the garden. Traditionally used to stop bleeding, reduce fevers, and support the immune system, it's an essential ally in any apothecary garden. With its powerful healing properties, Yarrow offers both physical and spiritual protection, making it a must-grow herb for every herbalist.

Plant Profile

- **Botanical Name:** Achillea millefolium
- **Common Names:** Soldier's Woundwort, Milfoil, Nosebleed Plant, Knight's Milfoil
- **Family:** Asteraceae (Daisy family)
- **Parts Used:** Aerial parts — flowers, leaves, stems (fresh or dried)
- **Taste:** Bitter, aromatic, slightly spicy
- **Energetics:** Drying, cooling (some say slightly warming internally)
- **Actions:** Astringent, styptic, vulnerary, diaphoretic, anti-inflammatory, antimicrobial, emmenagogue

Botanical Description

Yarrow is a hardy perennial with feathery, fern-like leaves and flat-topped clusters of tiny white to pink flowers. It grows wild in meadows, roadsides, and gardens, and has been used in traditional medicine across many cultures for centuries. The plant is named after Achilles, the Greek warrior who is said to have used Yarrow to treat his soldiers' wounds.

Grow Tip: Yarrow is drought-tolerant and hardy. It prefers poor soil and full sun.

Medicinal Uses

1. Wound Healing & First Aid

- Acts as a styptic (stops bleeding)
- Antiseptic and vulnerary (heals tissue)
- Use fresh or dried on cuts, nosebleeds, scrapes, bruises

2. Fever & Cold Support

- **Diaphoretic:** helps the body sweat out fevers
- Often blended with elderflower and peppermint as a classic cold & flu tea

3. Reproductive Support

- Helps bring on delayed menstruation
- Eases menstrual cramps and supports pelvic circulation
- Often used in teas or sitz baths for postpartum care

4. Gut & Liver Health

- Bitter compounds stimulate digestion and bile flow
- Calms intestinal spasms and supports liver detox

Traditional & Folk Uses

- Carried into battle as a first-aid herb for centuries
- Used to stop bleeding and draw out infection—even on the battlefield
- Believed to protect against evil, illness, and negative energy
- Used in divination and dream work (e.g. "Yarrow stalk" I Ching readings in China)
- Associated with balance, boundaries, and transitions

Magical & Energetic Associations

- **Element:** Water & Air
- **Planet:** Venus & Mars (protection and healing)
- **Chakras:** Root & Solar Plexus

— Used in protection, divination, energetic boundaries, and heart healing

— Said to close spiritual wounds and strengthen energetic sovereignty

— Worn during rituals to guard the spirit and clarify the mind

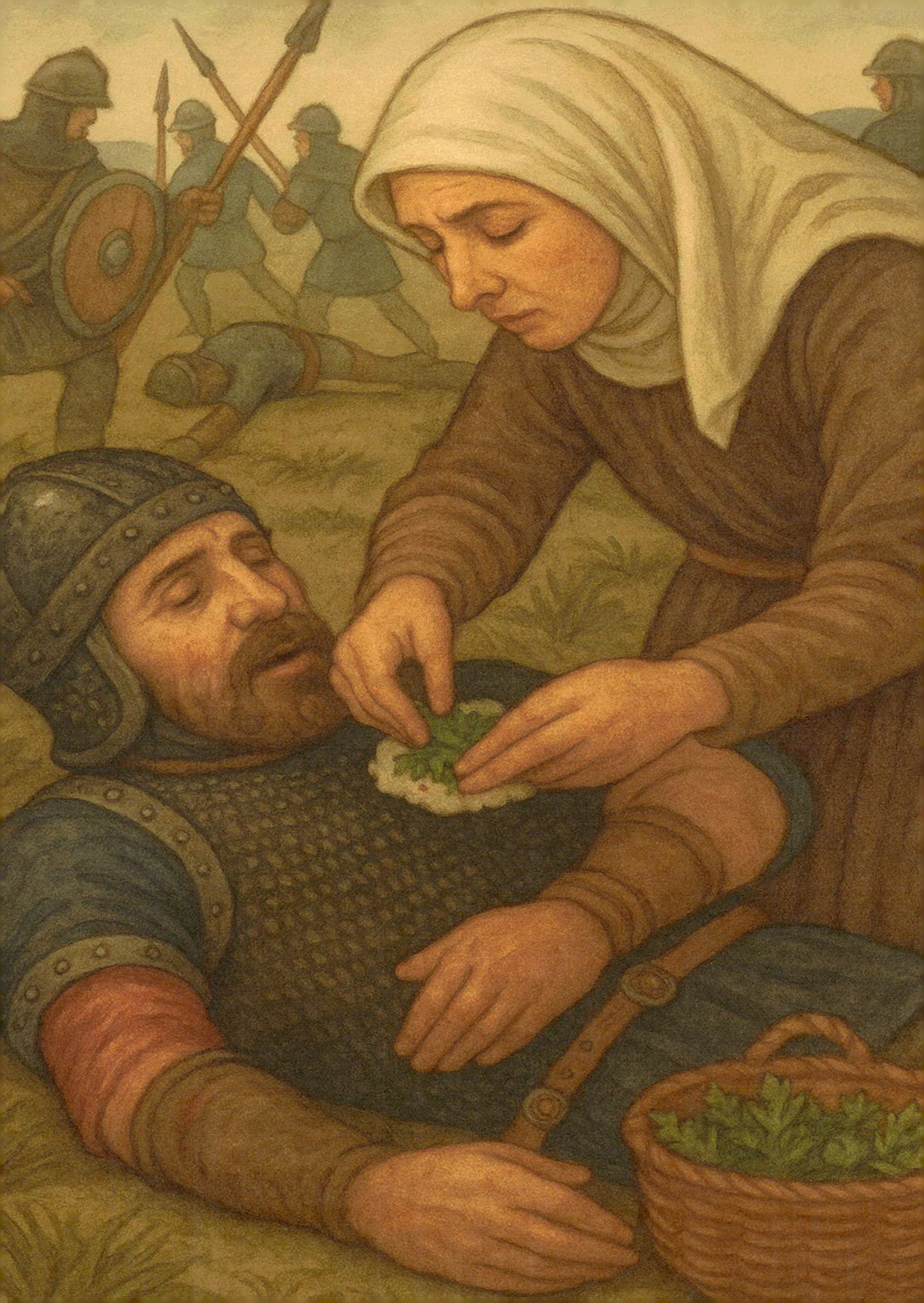

How to Use Yarrow

Tea (Infusion)

- 1–2 tsp dried herb per 8 oz water
- Steep covered for 10–15 minutes
- Use for colds, fevers, menstrual cramps, or digestion
- 1:5 in alcohol (40–50%)
- Dose: 20–40 drops, 2–3x/day

Poultice / Compress

- Chew fresh leaves or mash with warm water; apply to wounds, bruises, or bites

Bath or Sitz Bath

- Add strong infusion to bath water for soothing skin, pelvic care, or energetic clearing

How to Grow Yarrow

Yarrow is a low-maintenance, resilient herb with feathery leaves and clusters of tiny flowers — typically white, pink, or yellow. It's prized for its wound-healing, fever-breaking, and energetic boundary-setting properties.

Growing Notes

- Perennial in zones 3–9
- Loves full sun and well-drained, even poor soil
- Spreads easily — divide clumps every few years
- Harvest flowers just before full bloom for the strongest medicinal effect
- Leaves can be harvested anytime during the growing season

Start from Seed

From Seed:

- **Indoors**: 6–8 weeks before last frost
- **Outdoors**: After all danger of frost has passed

Steps:

1. Fill seed trays with moist, well-draining seed-starting mix.
2. Surface sow—do not bury! Yarrow needs light to germinate.
3. Mist gently to keep soil moist.
4. Keep warm in a sunny spot.
5. Germination typically takes 10–14 days.

How to Sprout Yarrow Seeds for Planting

You'll Need:

- Yarrow seeds
- Seed-starting mix (light and well-draining)
- Seed tray or small pots
- Spray bottle or gentle watering can
- Bright window or grow lights

Step-by-Step Instructions

1. Start indoors 6–8 weeks before last frost.
2. Fill trays with moist seed-starting mix (don't overpack).
3. Surface sow the seeds—press gently into the soil.
4. Mist gently and keep the soil moist but not soggy.
5. Keep warm and bright (ideal temperature: 65–70°F).
6. Germination typically occurs in 10–14 days.
7. Thin seedlings once they have 2–3 sets of true leaves.

After Sprouting

- Harden off before transplanting outdoors.
- Plant in full sun, spacing plants 12–24 inches apart.
- Water regularly at first, then taper off—Yarrow is drought-tolerant once established.

Can You Eat Yarrow Sprouts?

Technically, yes, but:

- The flavor is bitter and medicinal.
- It's better to wait until the flowers and leaves are mature for full healing potency.

Yarrow Herbal Tea Sipping Chart

Form	Amount per 8oz Water	Steeping Time	Best for
Fresh Petals	1 small handful (chopped)	10–15 minutes	Fever support, immune boost, stimulating digestion
Dried Petals	1–2 teaspoons	10–15 minutes	Menstrual regulation, mild fevers
Strong Infusion	1–2 tsp dried or double fresh	Steep 4–8 hours (covered)	Acute symptoms, fever, heavy menstruation, wound healing (internal)
Cold Brew	1 tbsp dried or fresh	Steep overnight in cool water	Cooling during heat or fever, gentle liver support, summer tonic

Benefits of Yarrow Tea

- Fever support
- Menstrual regulation
- Digestive aid
- Circulatory support
- Wound and skin healing (from within)

Safety of Yarrow by Age Group

Infants (Under 1 Year)

- Not recommended for internal use.
- Yarrow is too stimulating and bitter for infants. Avoid in teas or tinctures.
- Always patch test and use diluted preparations externally.

Children (1–6 Years) – External Only

- Use only externally (such as in diluted salves or bath soaks) and in small amounts.

Children (7–12 Years) – Topical + Mild Internal Use

- May use mild teas or external preparations under guidance.
- Introduce slowly and watch for allergic reactions, especially in those with ragweed or Asteraceae family sensitivities.

Teens & Adults

- Generally safe for most people in moderate doses.
- It can be used internally (tea, tincture, capsules) and externally.
- Avoid high doses during menstruation unless intentionally used for its uterine effects.

Elderly

Typically well-tolerated but monitor for medication interactions (especially blood thinners). Adjust dosage for sensitivity.

When to Use Caution

- Avoid internal use—Yarrow is an emmenagogue (stimulates uterine activity) and may not be safe during pregnancy.
- External use in low amounts (e.g., in a sitz bath) is generally fine.
- Yarrow is in the Asteraceae family—those with ragweed allergies should use with caution and perform a patch test before topical use.

YARROW NOTES

Personal Experiences

Preparations Tried

Favorite Uses

Blends / Parings

Harvest Notes

Other thoughts

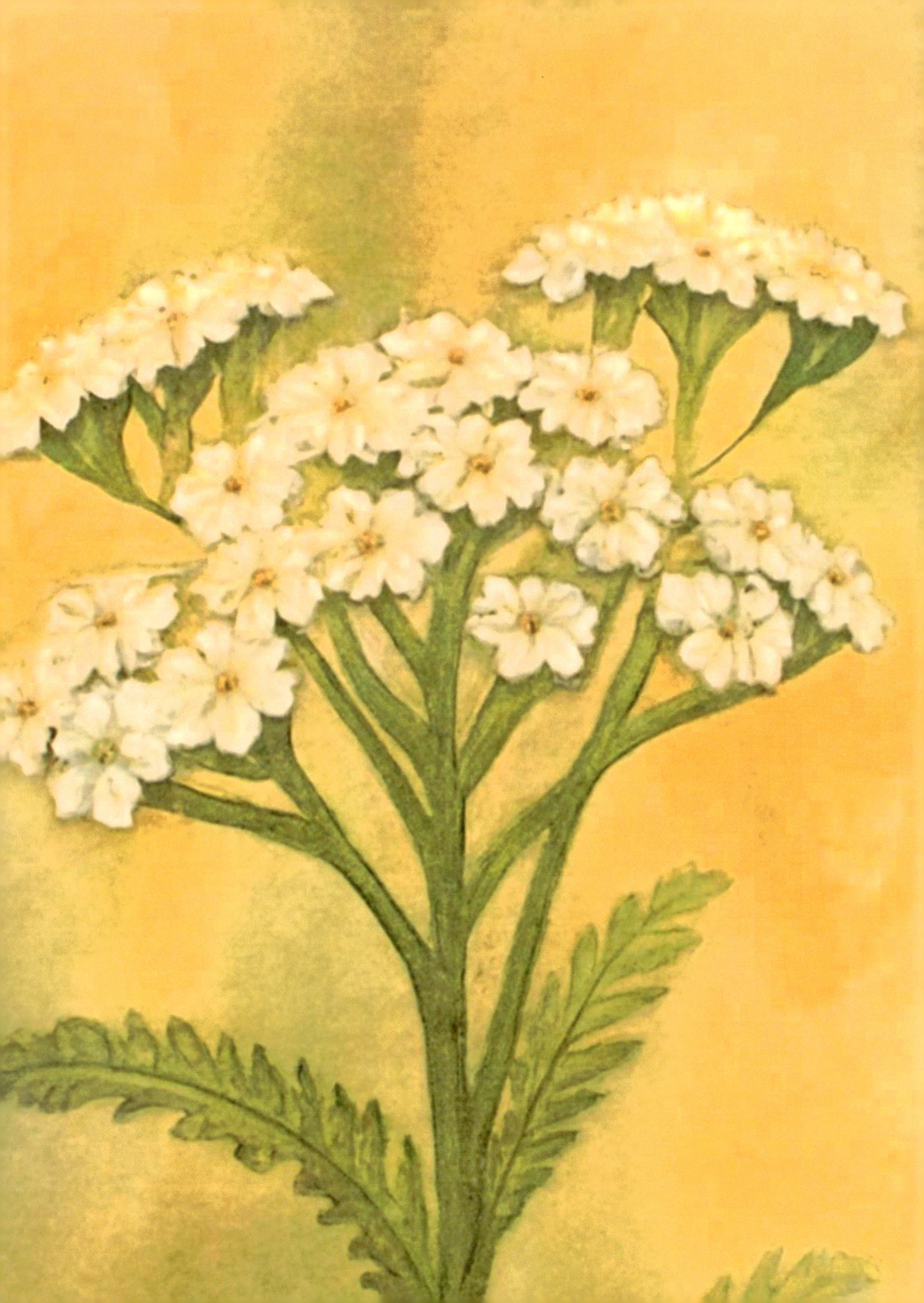

The Tale of Yarrow: The Warrior's Woundwort

In the days of old, when the world was wild and the gods walked among men, there lived a warrior named Achilles. He was fierce and near invincible, trained by the wise centaur Chiron, who taught him not only the art of war but also the secret knowledge of healing herbs.

Before Achilles went to battle in the great Trojan War, Chiron gave him a gift—not a weapon, but a humble plant with feathery leaves and clusters of white blooms. "This," said Chiron, "is Yarrow, the warrior's herb. It will stop blood, close wounds, and protect the body as surely as your shield."

Achilles carried it into battle, using it to treat his soldiers' wounds. Wherever he pressed its leaves to torn skin, the bleeding ceased. It was said that no herb was more powerful in stopping blood than this one, and for that, it became known as Achillea in his honor.

But Yarrow's power was not only for the battlefield.

In the villages, wise women and healers also used it—for fevers, grieving hearts, divination, and love spells. It was thrown into fires for protection, tucked under pillows to dream of one's future love, and planted at the edges of gardens to mark sacred boundaries.

Yarrow Whispers

Be soft as a feather, and sharp as a blade.
Protect what is sacred.
Heal what is broken.

NETTLE

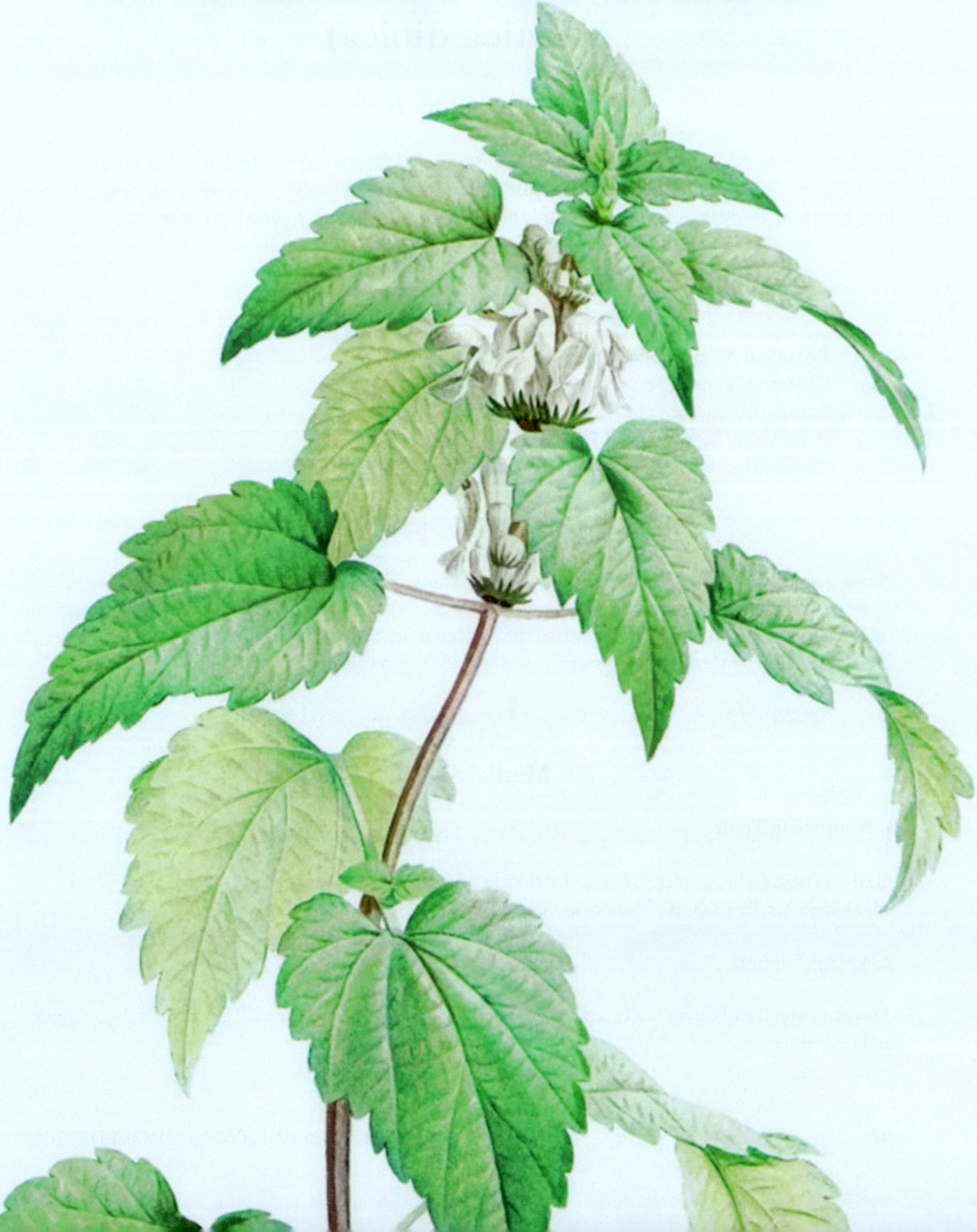

Nettle
(Urtica dioica)

Why Grow It?

Nettle is one of the most nourishing plants you can grow, often overlooked for its sting but beloved by herbalists for its strength. Packed with iron, calcium, and deep green vitality, nettle supports energy, allergies, joint health, and glowing skin from the inside out. It thrives in rich soil, returns year after year, and offers a powerful gift in every leaf. Once you know how to harvest her wisely, nettle becomes a lifelong ally.

Plant Profile

- **Botanical Name:** Urtica dioica
- **Common Names**: Stinging nettle, wild spinach
- **Family**: Urticaceae
- **Parts Used**: Leaves, stems, flowers, roots, seed
- **Taste:** Salty and sweet

Botanical Description

Nettle is a hardy perennial herb known for its fierce sting and remarkable benefits. It grows 2–4 feet tall with square stems and sharply serrated, deep green leaves. Both stems and leaves are covered in tiny stinging hairs (trichomes) that deliver a sharp, tingling sensation when touched fresh. The plant produces small, greenish flowers in drooping clusters during summer and spreads vigorously via underground rhizomes.

Grow Tip: Prefers partial shade to full sun and rich, moist, well-drained soil.

Medicinal Uses

1. Nourishing Tonic

Ideal for those feeling depleted, fatigued, or low in minerals. Long infusions are especially helpful for rebuilding after illness, heavy menstruation, or burnout.

2. Allergy Support

Acts as a natural antihistamine. Taken regularly before allergy season, nettle may reduce sneezing, itching, and sinus irritation.

3. Urinary & Kidney Health

A mild diuretic, nettle promotes healthy fluid elimination and can assist with UTIs, edema, or gout by reducing uric acid levels.

4. Iron-Rich & Blood Building

Nettle's combination of iron and vitamin C makes it excellent for anemia and those with heavy cycles or low energy.

5. Hair, Skin & Joint Health

Used both internally and topically to support hair growth, clearer skin, stronger nails, and relieve arthritic inflammation.

Traditional & Folk Uses

- Spring tonic, food as medicine
- Blood builder
- Strength restorer
- Allergy relief
- Joint & Muscle aches
- Nettle was used in ritual "urtication"—brushing fresh nettles on aching joints to bring blood flow and healing
- Urinary & kidney support
- Postpartum and menstrual support

Magical & Energetic Associations

- **Element:** Fire
- **Planet:** Mars
- **Chakra:** Root & Solar Plexus
- **Energy:** Protective, cleansing, strengthening, awakening

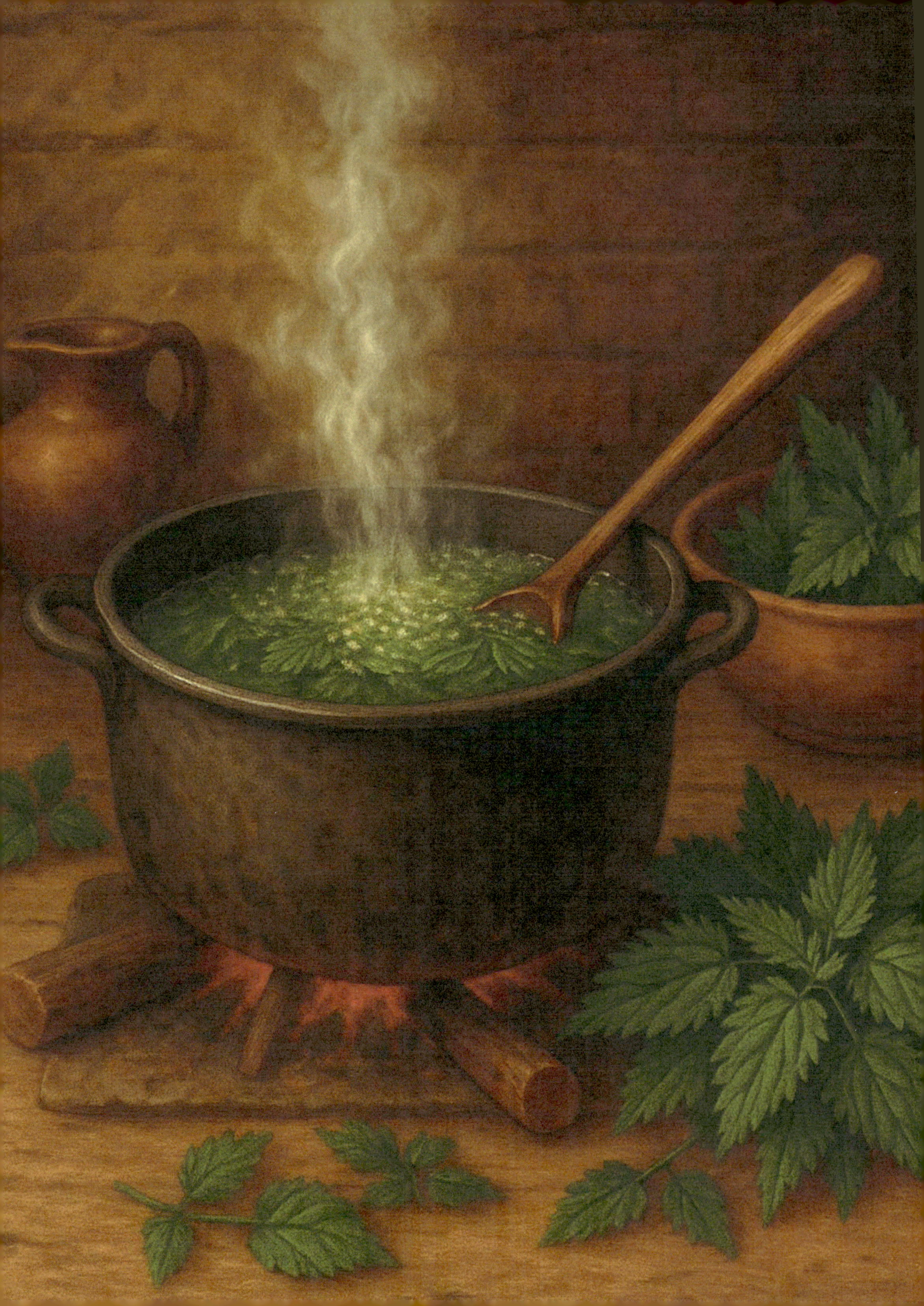

How to Use Nettle

Infusion (Tea)

- 1–2 tsp dried leaves per 8oz of water
- Steep 10–15 minutes, covered
- Drink for lymph, digestion, or inflammation

Edible

- Fresh leaves steamed or sautéed like spinach
- Use in soups, stews, nettle pesto
- Dry and crush into a sea

Oil Infusion

- Soak dried nettle in oil for 4-6 weeks, use on joints or scalp

Hair Rinse

- Brew a strong tea, allow to cool, pour over scalp to support growth and soothe inflammation

Tincture

Great for allergy relief, joint support

How to Grow Nettle

Nettle is a low-maintenance, resilient herb that thrives in rich soil and partial shade. It's prized for its wound-healing, mineral-rich leaves and is incredibly easy to grow with the right care.

Growing Notes

- Perennial in zones 3–9
- Loves full sun and well-drained, even poor soil
- Spreads easily—divide clumps every few years
- Harvest flowers just before full bloom for strongest medicinal effect
- Leaves can be harvested anytime during the growing season

Start from Seed

From Seed

- **Indoors**: 6–8 weeks before last frost
- **Outdoors:** After all danger of frost has passed

Steps:

- Fill seed trays with moist, well-draining seed-starting mix.
- Surface sow—do not bury! Nettle needs light to germinate.
- Mist gently to keep soil moist.
- Keep warm in a sunny spot.
- Germination typically takes 10–14 days.

How to Sprout Nettle Seeds for Planting

You'll Need

- Nettle seeds
- Seed-starting mix (light and well-draining)
- Seed tray or small pots
- Spray bottle or gentle watering can
- Bright window or grow lights

Step-by-Step Instructions

- Start indoors 6–8 weeks before last frost.
- Fill trays with moist seed-starting mix (don't overpack).
- Surface sow the seeds—press gently into the soil.
- Mist gently and keep the soil moist but not soggy.
- Keep warm and bright (ideal temperature: 65–70°F).
- Germination typically occurs in 10–14 days.
- Thin seedlings once they have 2–3 sets of true leaves.

After Sprouting

- Harden off before transplanting outdoors.
- Plant in full sun, spacing plants 12–24 inches apart.
- Water regularly at first, then taper off—Nettle is drought-tolerant once established.

Can You Eat Nettle Sprouts?

Technically, yes, but:

- The flavor is bitter and medicinal.
- It's better to wait until the flowers and leaves are mature for full healing potency.

Nettle Herbal Tea Sipping Chart

Form	Amount per 8oz Water	Steeping Time	Best for
Fresh Petals	1.5 – 2 tsp chopped	8-10 minutes	Spring sipping, light nourishment
Dried Petals	1 tsp	10-15 minutes	Daily tonic, allergy support, gentle detox
Strong Infusion	1 oz (1 cup)	4-8 hours or overnight	Mineral boost, postpartum, adrenal support
Cold Brew	1.5–2 Tbsp per quart	6-12 hours (fridge)	Summer sipping hydration, gentle detox

Benefits of Nettle Tea

- Rich in minerals and vitamins
- Natural allergy relief
- Supports blood & circulation
- Kidney & urinary support
- Strengthens hair, skin, and nails
- Anti-inflammatory & joint comfort
- Gentle daily tonic

Safety of Nettle by Age Group

Infants (Under 1 Year)

- Not recommended for internal use.
- Their kidneys and systems are still developing, and even mild herbal infusions may be too stimulating. Avoid internal use, and do not apply topically unless guided by a pediatric herbalist.

Toddlers (1–3 Years)

Use with extreme caution. While a very dilute nettle tea (1–2 minute steep) is sometimes used in pediatric formulas, it's best reserved for experienced practitioners. Topical use is also risky due to nettle's stinging hairs—avoid wild nettle contact.

Children (4–12 Years)

Nettle can be introduced in very mild infusions (¼–½ tsp dried nettle per cup, steeped briefly). It's a great source of gentle minerals and can support seasonal allergies or energy in kids. Avoid concentrated infusions or tinctures without guidance. Always strain well to remove stinging hairs.

Teens (13–17 Years)

Safe in moderate amounts. Teens can enjoy standard nettle tea (1 tsp dried per cup, 10–15 min steep) to support energy, skin clarity, and hormonal balance. Nettle is especially helpful for active teens with joint soreness or fatigue. Infusions (1 oz to 1 qt water) can be used under supervision.

Adults (18–64 Years)

Nettle is considered very safe and deeply nourishing for adults. Daily tea or strong infusions can support iron levels, reduce inflammation, and restore energy. However, it may act as a diuretic, so those with low blood pressure or electrolyte imbalances should start slowly. Long-term use may require mineral replenishment from food or companion herbs like oat straw or red clover.

Pregnancy

Nettle is often used in pregnancy teas as a source of gentle minerals and iron. However, it should be used with care, especially early in pregnancy, due to its mildly stimulating effect on the uterus. Always use under the guidance of a midwife or herbalist. Tea is typically safe in moderate amounts after the first trimester.

Breastfeeding

Nettle can help support milk production and maternal energy. It's often included in lactation blends and mineral-rich postpartum teas. Mild daily tea is considered safe, but watch for increased urination or any signs of baby sensitivity (rare).

Elders (65+)

Nettle is excellent for elders when used in moderation. It supports joint health, circulation, and bone strength—but its diuretic action means it should be used carefully if someone is on medications for blood pressure, fluid retention, or kidney health. Start with small doses and monitor hydration levels.

NETTLE NOTES

Personal Experiences

Preparations Tried

Favorite Uses

Blends / Parings

Harvest Notes

Other thoughts

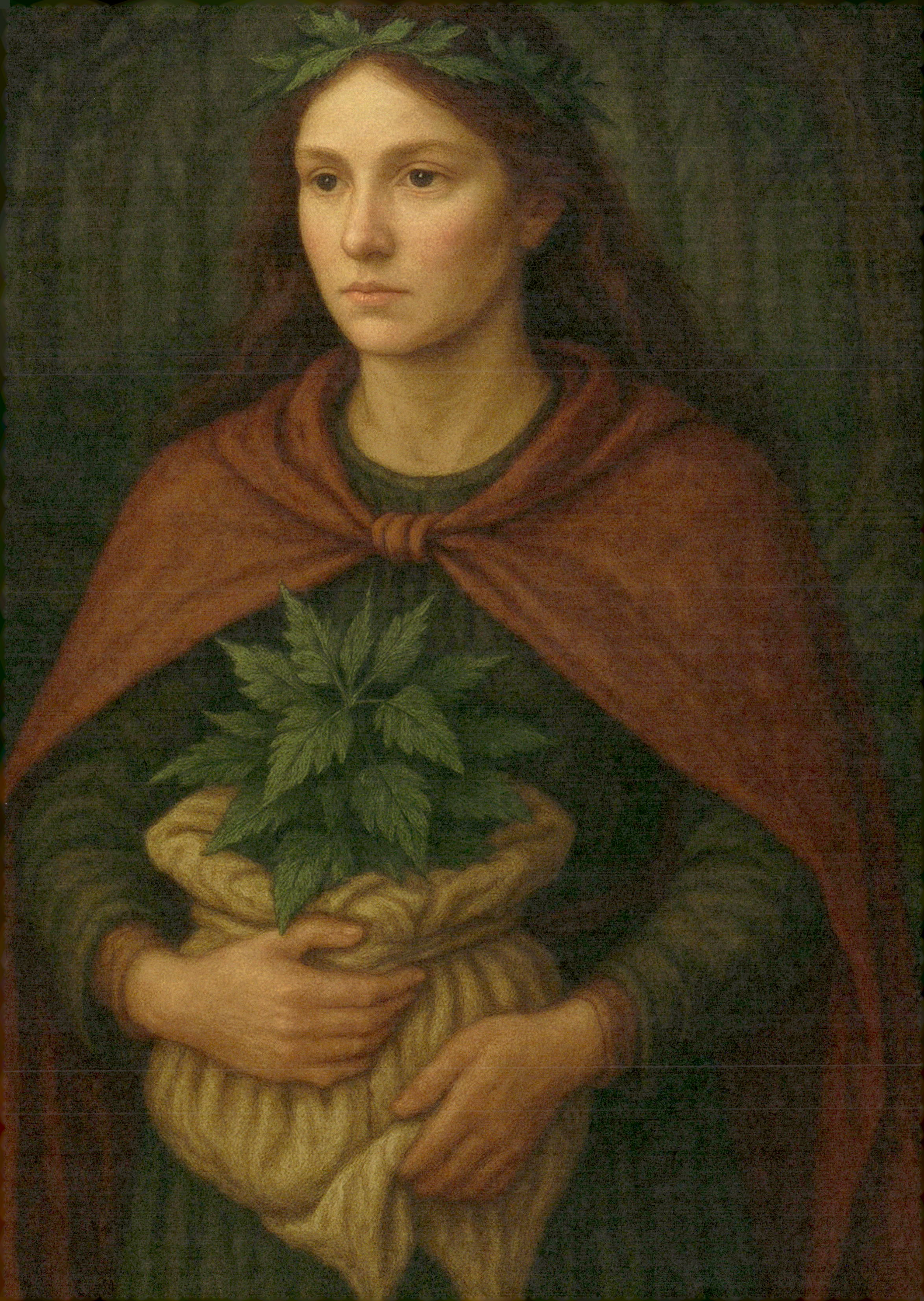

Nettle: The Sister's Redemption

Long ago, in a kingdom surrounded by wild woods, there lived eleven princes and one princess. They were all children of a wise and kind queen. But when the queen passed, the king was bewitched by a jealous sorceress who feared the children's light. With dark magic, she turned the princes into swans and cast the princess, Elise, into exile.

Years passed. One day, Elise wandered deep into the forest where an old wise woman revealed a way to break the curse:

She must gather the stinging nettles. It grew in graveyards and on forgotten hills. She would then spin them into thread and weave eleven shirts—one for each brother. Only then could they be freed. But there was one more condition:

She must do this in complete silence, not uttering a word, even if it cost her life.

Elise suffered terribly. Her hands bled from the nettle's sting. Villagers mocked her as she worked, and the king of a nearby land, enchanted by her beauty, took her as his bride. But still, she never spoke. She spun and wove in secret.

Just as the last shirt was finished, Elise was accused of witchcraft and sentenced to burn at the stake. But as the fire was lit, she threw the nettle shirts over the swans that circled overhead. The spell broke. Her brothers returned to human form. She had completed her task, and her silence ended.

She was cleared of all charges, and the land rejoiced.

Nettle Teaches

Not all that stings is cruel. Some trials come to awaken our strength and transform pain into power.

ECHINACEA

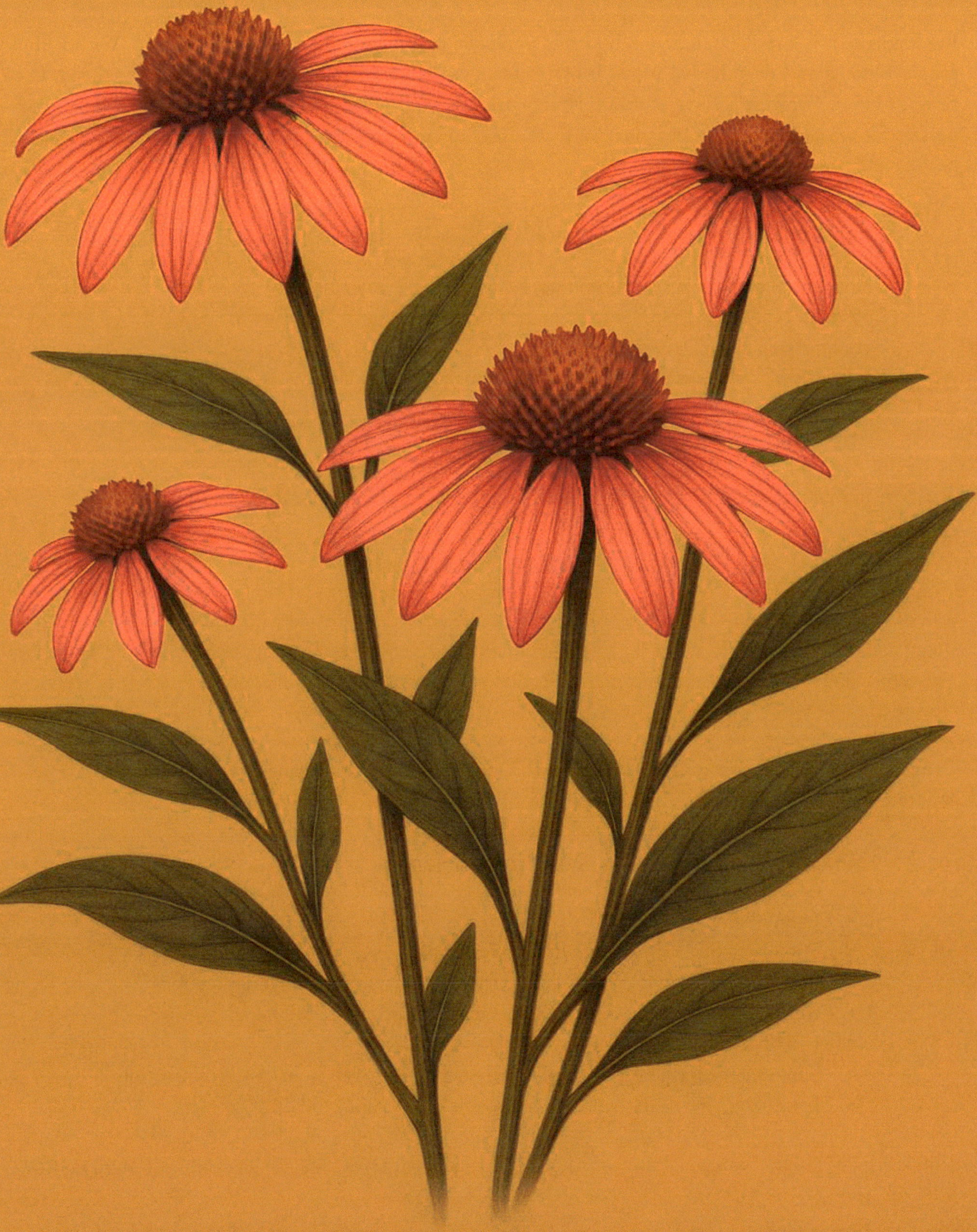

Echinacea
(Urtica dioica)

Why Grow It?

In summary, it is a resilient, immune-boosting perennial that belongs in every home garden. With its bold purple blooms and deep herbal roots, it offers beauty, pollinator support, and powerful medicine from flower to root. Growing echinacea means having natural, whole-plant immune support at your fingertips—perfect for teas, tinctures, and seasonal wellness. Easy to grow and rich in tradition, echinacea brings both healing and heart to your herbal practice.

Plant Profile

- **Botanical Name**: Echinacea purpurea, E. angustifolia, E. pallida
- **Common Names**: Purple Coneflower, Snakeroot, American Coneflower
- **Family:** Asteraceae (Daisy family)
- **Parts Used:** Root, flower, seed, and sometimes leaves
- **Taste:** Pungent, slightly sweet, tingling
- **Energetics:** Cooling, drying

Actions: Immune stimulant, lymphatic, anti-inflammatory, antimicrobial, alterative

Botanical Description

Echinacea is a hardy, sun-loving perennial native to the central and eastern United States. It features tall stems with distinctive pink-purple petals and spiny, cone-shaped centers that attract bees and butterflies. The genus name Echinacea comes from the Greek word echinos, meaning hedgehog, referring to its prickly seed head.

Grow Tip: Prefers full sun and well-drained soil. Once established, it's drought-tolerant and low maintenance.

Medicinal Uses

- Immune Support
- Stimulates the body's innate immune response
- Best used at the first sign of illness, especially respiratory or viral infections
- Activates macrophages and increases white blood cell activity
- Lymphatic & Detoxifying
- Supports the lymphatic system — reduces swollen glands, helps clear infection
- Encourages gentle detoxification through lymph, skin, and urinary tract

- Anti-inflammatory & Antimicrobial
- Used for wound healing, sore throats, gum infections, and abscesses
- Can be applied as a wash or compress for minor cuts and skin irritations

Preventative & Short-Term Use

Not a daily tonic herb — best used for acute care or short seasonal support

Traditional & Folk Uses

- Used by Indigenous peoples of North America for snake bites, toothaches, infections, and wounds
- Nicknamed "snakeroot" for its ability to pull infection and poison from the body
- Early settlers adopted it as a panacea for fevers, colds, and general malaise
- Carried in medicine bundles or burned in ceremonies for spiritual purification and immunity
- Believed to strengthen the body's defenses and awaken inner vitality

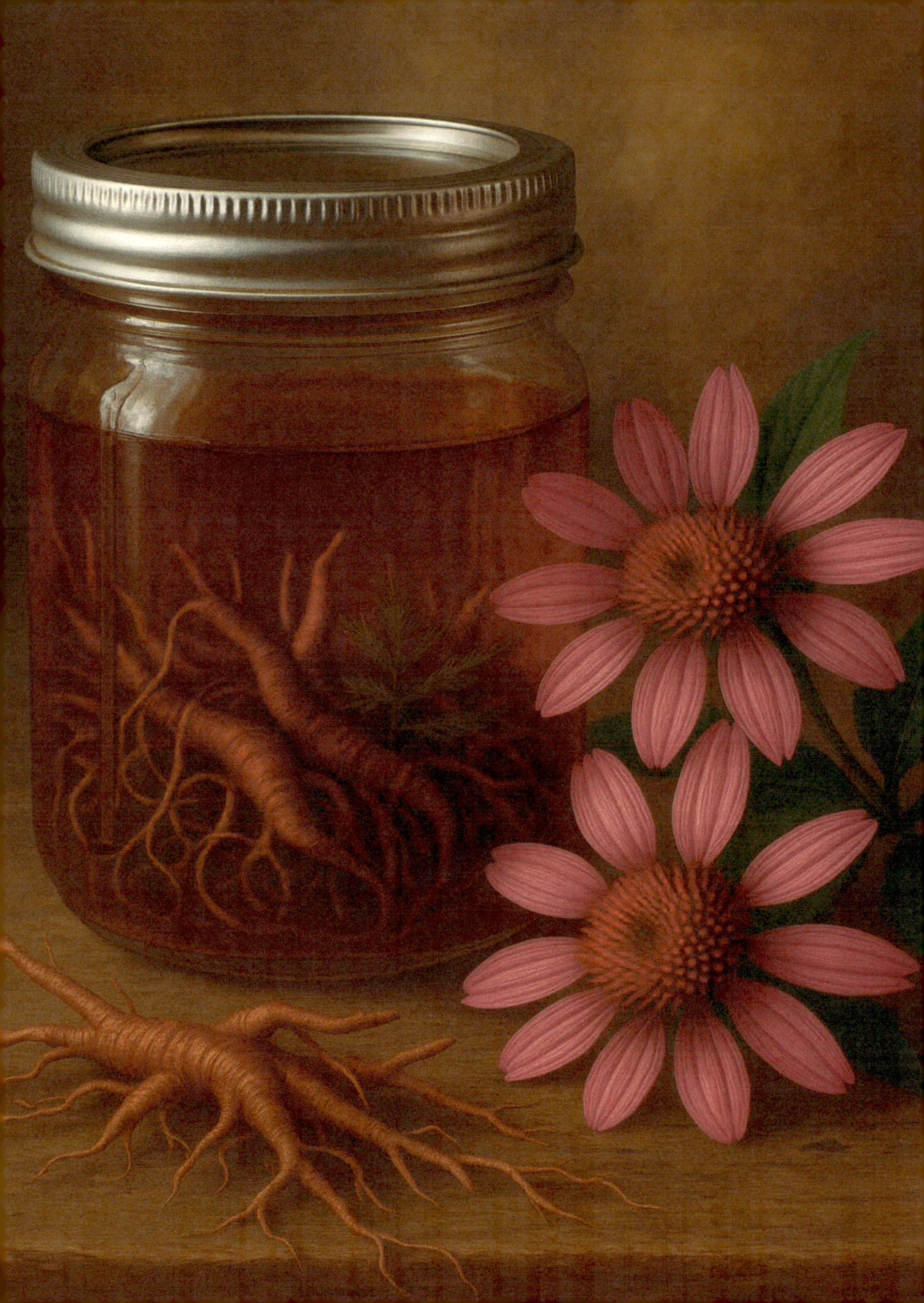

Magical & Energetic Associations

- **Element:** Earth & Fire
- **Planet:** Mars
- **Chakra:** Root

— Used in spells and charms for: Protection, boundary-setting, healing, and vitality
Said to: Strengthen the aura and repel negative energy or illness

How to Use Echinacea

1. **Tincture**

    - Use root or whole plant (1:5 ratio in 50–60% alcohol)
    - Dose: 30–60 drops up to 3x/day at onset of illness
    - For prevention: 10–30 drops 1x/day for 1–2 weeks during high-risk times

2. **Tea (Decoction)**

    - Simmer 1 tsp of dried root in 1 cup water for 15–20 minutes
    - Add herbs like ginger, elderflower, or peppermint for flu blends

3. **Topical Use**

    - Strong tea or tincture diluted in water as a wound wash or gargle
    - Infused oil or salve (less common, but possible for skin infections)

How to Grow Echinacea

Echinacea is a hardy, drought-tolerant perennial known for its immune-supportive roots and vibrant flowers. Beloved by herbalists, pollinators, and garden witches alike, it's a must-have for both beauty and medicine.

Growing Notes

- Perennial in zones 3–9
- Prefers full sun and well-drained soil
- Drought-tolerant once established
- Flowers bloom in late summer — harvest roots in the fall of year 2+ for strongest potency
- Flowers also usable for mild tea blends and aesthetic value
- Start from Seed

Cold Stratify Seeds for Best Germination: Place in damp sand or paper towel in the fridge for 2–4 weeks

Sow Indoors

- 8–10 weeks before last frost
- Press seeds lightly into the soil — they need light to sprout
- Keep moist and warm (germination in 10–21 days)
- Transplant outdoors after danger of frost has passed

Direct Sow (Spring or Fall)

- Sow seeds in fall or early spring after natural cold exposure
- Germination occurs as temperatures warm

Harvesting

- Leaves & Flowers
- Harvest flowers when fully open (late summer)
- Leaves can be harvested any time in year 1+
- Use in teas, tinctures, and salves

Roots

- Wait until year 3 or later to dig for root harvest
- Best harvested in fall, after plant has gone dormant
- Wash, chop, and dry or tincture immediately
- Companion Plant & Pollinator Magnet
- Attracts bees, butterflies, and beneficial insects
- Pairs beautifully with yarrow, bee balm, calendula, and lemon balm

Perennial Zones

- Hardy in zones 3–9
- Cut back stems in late fall or early spring
- Mulch lightly in winter in northern climates

Apothecary Use

- Root is used for immune stimulation and lymphatic support
- Flowers and leaves can be used for gentler cold & flu support
- Combine with elderflower, peppermint, or lemon balm in classic wellness blends

Sprouting Echinacea: The Immune Warrior in Miniature

Echinacea is best known for its immune-supporting roots and vibrant purple flowers—but did you know the young sprouts also hold gentle medicinal magic?

Sprouting echinacea gives you a tender, nutrient-rich version of the plant in just days. While it won't replace mature root or flower preparations for deep immune work, echinacea sprouts offer a fresh, green way to support wellness—especially when added to food or used in gentle tea infusions.

How to Sprout Echinacea Seeds

Materials

- Organic echinacea seeds (look for Echinacea purpurea)
- Wide-mouth jar or sprouting tray
- Mesh lid or cheesecloth
- Clean water

Steps

- Soak seeds in cool water for 4–6 hours. Drain and rinse.
- Place in your sprouting jar or tray, draining well to avoid mold.
- Rinse and drain twice daily.
- Sprouts typically emerge in 3–5 days.
- Harvest when they're ½–1 inch long, with tiny green tips.

Tip: Echinacea seeds can be slow to sprout and may need cooler temperatures. Be patient—they're worth it!

Uses for Echinacea Sprouts

- Immune-supporting garnish: Add to salads, grain bowls, or sandwiches for a bitter-green boost.
- Mild infusion: Steep a small handful (1–2 tsp) in hot water for 5–7 minutes for a gentle immune tonic.
- Tincture base: Use young sprouts for a unique early-season echinacea tincture (combine with older roots later).
- Smoothie booster: Blend into green smoothies to layer in mild, earthy immune support.

Echinacea Herbal Tea Sipping Chart

Form	Amount per 8oz Water	Steeping Time	Best for
Fresh leaves or flowers	1 handful (chopped)	10-15 minutes	Earthy, mildly floral
Fresh leaves or flowers	1-2 teaspoons (chopped)	15-20 minutes	Strong tingling earthy
Strong Infusion	1 Tbsp dried root	Simmer 4-8 hours	Acute symptoms, short-term immune boost
Cold brew	1 tbsp dried or fresh	Steep 8-12 hours in cool water	Summer immune tonic, cooling support, daily wellness brew

Benefits of Echinacea Tea

- Immune activation
- Throat and upper respiratory relief
- Lymphatic support
- Wound healing (from within)
- Emotional fortitude

Safety of Echinacea by Age Group

Infants (Under 1 Year)

- Echinacea is not recommended due to their still-developing immune and digestive systems

Children (1–12 Years)

- Should be limited to very small doses and only when truly needed—such as at the onset of a cold—and preferably under the guidance of a qualified herbalist or pediatrician.

Teens & Adults

- Echinacea is generally well-tolerated and often used at the first sign of illness or to support recovery.

Elderly

- Echinacea can be beneficial for immune modulation but may interact with immune-related medications or conditions.

Safety & Cautions

- Generally considered safe for short-term use
- May cause rare allergic reactions in those sensitive to the Asteraceae family
- Not recommended for long-term use (more than 6–8 weeks) or autoimmune conditions without guidance
- Not ideal during pregnancy unless directed by a practitioner, as research is limited though no major risks have been identified.

ECHINACEA NOTES

Personal Experiences

Preparations Tried

Favorite Uses

Blends / Parings

Harvest Notes

Other thoughts

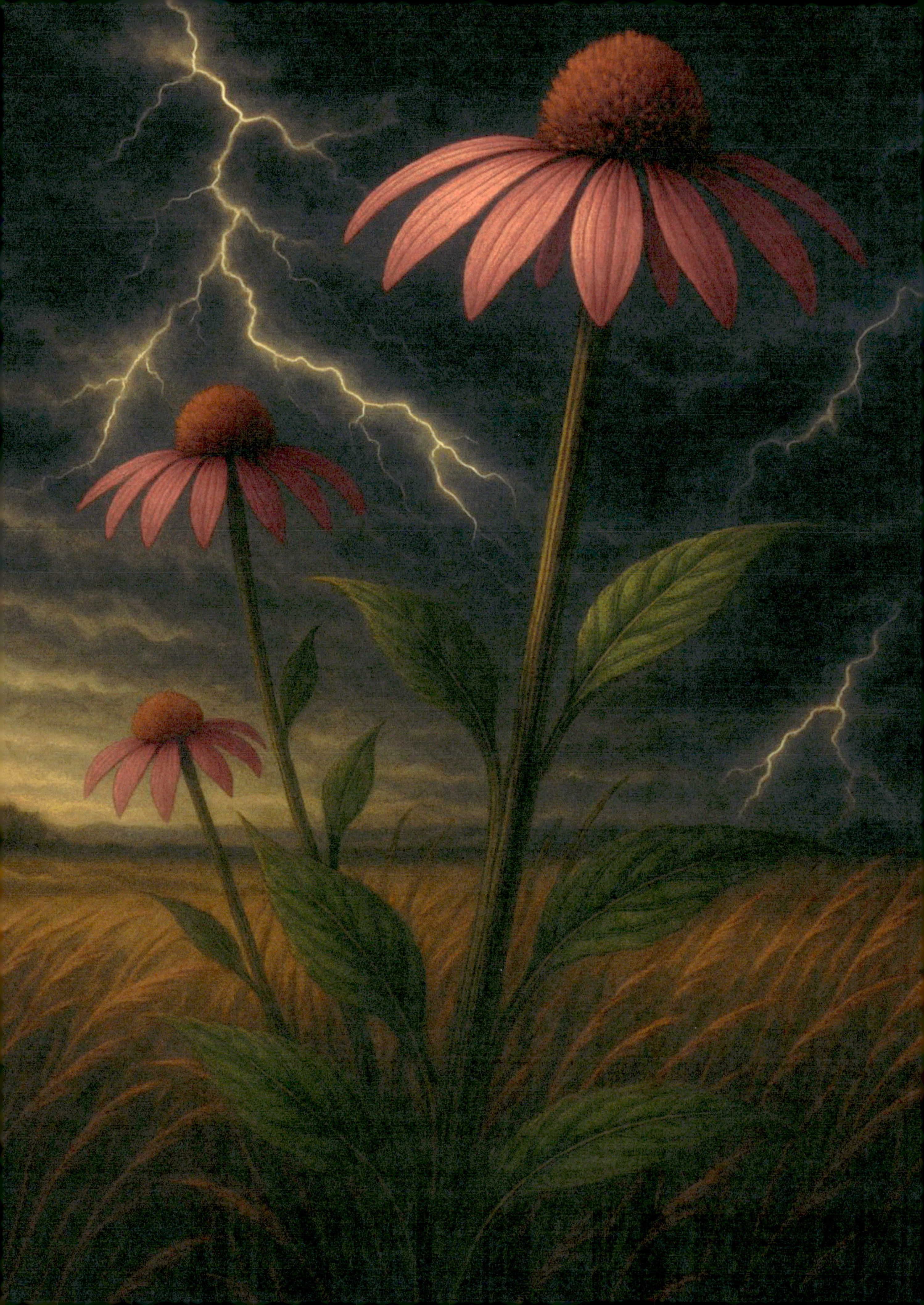

Echinacea: The Flower That Fought the Storm

In the wide, open prairies where the sky stretches and thunder sings through the hills, the people watched the horizon. A great sickness was coming; a storm not of rain or wind, but of illness that left the strong weak and the wise afraid.

The healers gathered beneath the sky and prayed to the Earth for help. For days, there was no answer. But then a child, quiet and often overlooked, wandered into the tall grasses at dawn. She did not cry out or ask for signs, she simply listened.

And there, glowing in the morning light, stood a flower she had never seen before. It was a purple cone rising from a sea of petals, like a warrior's shield beneath the sun. Bees danced over it, and a breeze carried its scent of deep, living earth.

The child dug its root gently, brought it to the elders, and said: "This flower stood while the others bent. Maybe it remembers how to fight."

The healers brewed the root into a strong tea and gave it to the sick. Day by day, those who drank it grew stronger. The flower became known as the Guardian of the People.

Echinacea whispers

Even in the storm, I stand tall. I do not break. I defend. I endure.

ROSEMARY

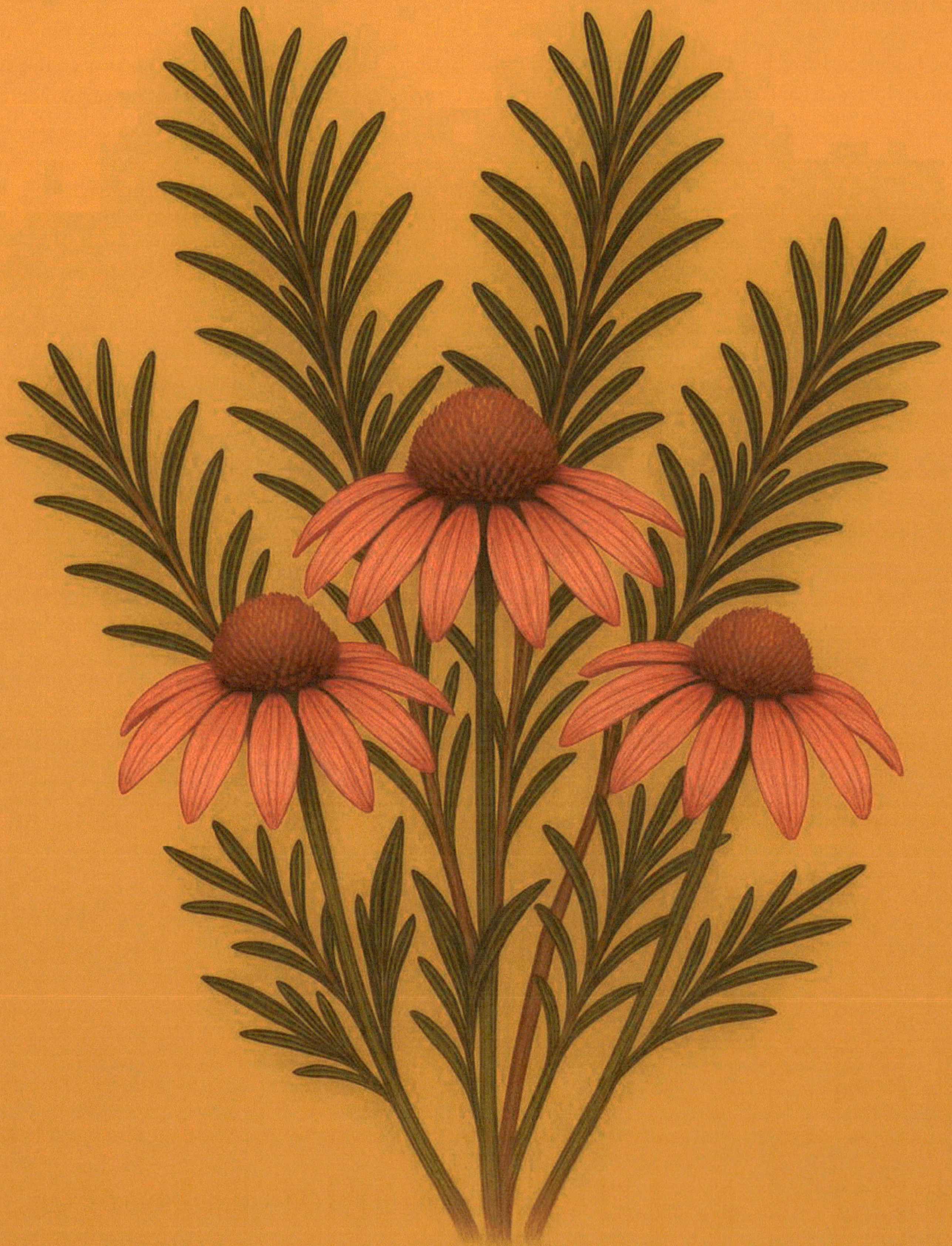

Rosemary (Salvia rosmarinus)

Why Grow It?

In summary, it's a resilient and versatile herb that deserves a place in every garden and kitchen. With its fragrant, evergreen needles and blue flowers, rosemary thrives in sun-drenched soil and offers year-round beauty. But beyond its visual charm, it's a powerful medicinal plant. Known to sharpen the mind, soothe digestion, uplift the spirit, and invigorate circulation, rosemary is a true ally. Brew it into tea, infuse it in oils, or simply run your hand over the fragrant leaves to enjoy its aromatic lift. Rosemary brings clarity, resilience, and tradition into your daily rituals.

Plant Profile

- **Botanical Name:** Salvia rosmarinus (formerly Rosmarinus officinalis)
- **Common Names:** Rosemary, dew of the sea
- **Family:** Lamiaceae (Mint family)
- **Parts Used:** Leaves, stems, flowers
- **Taste:** Pungent, piney, slightly bitter
- **Energetics:** Warming, drying
- **Actions:** Stimulant, circulatory tonic, nervine, antimicrobial, memory-enhancing

Botanical Description

Rosemary is a woody, evergreen shrub with needle-like aromatic leaves and delicate blue, purple, or white flowers. Native to the Mediterranean, it thrives in dry, sunny places and has been celebrated for its culinary and medicinal properties for thousands of years. It is also a symbol of remembrance, purification, and protection.

Grow Tip: Rosemary thrives in full sun and well-drained soil. It's drought-tolerant once established, making it a great low-maintenance option.

Medicinal Uses

1. **Memory + Mental Clarity**

    - Enhances focus, cognition, and circulation to the brain
    - Traditionally burned or infused for clarity in study or ritual

2. **Circulation + Warmth**

    - Warms cold hands and feet
    - Stimulates blood flow and eases mild pain or stiffness when used topically

3. **Antimicrobial + Antioxidant**

    - Powerful against bacteria and viruses
    - Used in cleansing sprays, oils, and natural preservatives

4. **Hair + Scalp Health**

    - Infused into oil or vinegar to promote hair growth, scalp stimulation, and shine

5. **Digestive Support**

    - Eases sluggish digestion and gas
    - Combats heaviness and bloating when added to meals or teas

Traditional & Folk Uses

- Burned to ward off illness and negative energy
- Used at funerals and weddings as a symbol of remembrance and fidelity
- Carried or worn for protection, courage, and purification

Magical & Energetic Associations

- **Element:** Fire
- **Planet:** Sun
- **Chakra:** Third Eye & Solar Plexus

— Used for memory, purification, protection, and clarity
— Hung in doorways or burned to bless and cleanse a home

How to Use Rosemary

1. **Tea**

    1 tsp dried or 1 tbsp fresh leaf per cup. Steep for 10-15 minutes (covered). Drink for clarity, digestion, or cold support

2. **Tincture**

    1:5 in 40-50% alcohol. Dose: 20-40 drops as needed

3. **Infused Oil**

    Use in salves, hair treatments, or massage blends

4. **Steam or Smoke**

    Great in facial steams for congestion. Burn for cleansing, focus, or ritual space clearing

How to Grow Rosemary

Rosemary is a sun-loving, aromatic evergreen. It thrives in dry, sunny places and is prized for its culinary use, medicinal properties, and spiritual significance.

Growing Notes:

- Perennial in zones 7–10 (grow as an annual or in containers in colder zones)
- Prefers full sun, dry to sandy soil, and excellent drainage
- Water deeply but infrequently
- Prune regularly to keep it bushy and avoid woodiness
- Can be propagated by cuttings in spring or fall

How to Grow from Cuttings (Easiest Method)

1. Take a 4–6 inch cutting from new, soft stem growth (not woody).
2. Strip lower leaves and place in water or damp potting mix.
3. Roots form in 2–4 weeks.
4. Transplant into pot or directly into the garden once rooted and stable.

How to Grow from Seed (Patience Required)

1. Start indoors 8–12 weeks before the last frost.
2. Use light, well-drained seed-starting mix.
3. Surface sow or lightly press in — rosemary needs light to germinate.
4. Keep warm (70-75°F) and moist.
5. Germination may take 2–4 weeks or longer.
6. Transplant when seedlings are 2–3 inches tall and sturdy.

Harvesting Tips

- Snip sprigs anytime once the plant is well-established (6–8 inches tall or more).
- Frequent trimming encourages bushy growth.
- For drying, harvest in the morning when oils are strong but the dew has lifted.

Overwintering

- Rosemary is a tender perennial in zones 7 and up. In colder climates, bring potted rosemary indoors before frost.
- Place in a sunny window and water sparingly. Outdoors, mulch heavily and shelter if overwintering in-ground.

How to Sprout Rosemary Seeds for Planting

Supplies

- Rosemary seeds
- Light, well-draining seed-starting mix
- Seed tray or shallow pots
- Clear humidity dome or plastic wrap (optional)
- Heat mat or warm location
- Grow light or sunny windowsill

Step-by-Step Instructions

1. Soak seeds overnight (this softens the tough seed coat and improves germination).
2. Prepare trays with moist seed-starting mix.
3. Surface sow seeds and lightly press into the soil. Do not bury them deeply — they need light to germinate.
4. Mist gently and cover with plastic to retain humidity. Keep moist but not wet.
5. Place in a warm spot. Ideal temperature: 70-80°F (21-27°C). A heat mat works wonders.
6. Germination may take 14 to 30 days (sometimes longer). Be patient!
7. Once sprouted, remove cover and place in bright light. Thin seedlings when they reach 2–3 inches tall.

After Sprouting

- Harden off before transplanting outdoors.
- Transplant to well-drained soil in full sun.
- Let the soil dry between waterings — rosemary is drought-tolerant once established.

Can You Eat Rosemary Sprouts?

Technically yes, but:

- They grow very slowly and are not typically eaten as microgreens.
- Rosemary is most valued when mature, as the leaves are rich in volatile oils and medicinal properties.

Rosemary Herbal Tea Sipping Chart

Form	Amount per 8oz water	Steeping Time	Best for
Fresh leaves	1.5 – 2 tsp	8–12 minutes	Headache relief, mood lifting
Dried leaves	1 tsp	5–10 minutes	Mental clarity, digestion
Strong Infusion	2 tsp dry or fresh	15+ minutes	Circulation, fatigue
Cold brew	—	6-12 hours (fridge)	Summer sipping, gentle uplift

Benefits of Rosemary Tea

- Cognitive clarity and memory support
- Circulation and anti-inflammatory
- Digestive aid and bloat relief
- Stress reduction and mood boosting
- Antioxidant and immune support

Safety of Rosemary by Age Group

Infants (Under 1 Year)

Rosemary should not be used internally for infants. Their systems are too delicate to handle rosemary's potent volatile oils.

Adults (18–64 years)

Rosemary is generally safe and beneficial for most adults. Standard doses of tea, tincture, infused oil, and culinary use are all appropriate. However, those with epilepsy, high blood pressure, or on medications such as blood thinners or diuretics should monitor closely and consult with a practitioner before using rosemary regularly or in concentrated form.

Pregnancy

While rosemary is generally safe in small culinary or tea amounts during pregnancy, concentrated forms (like tincture or essential oil) should be avoided. Rosemary is known to stimulate uterine activity in high doses, so it's wise to limit intake to an occasional, mild tea and avoid any form that could be too stimulating.

Breastfeeding

Rosemary tea and food use are typically safe while breastfeeding. There are no known concerns when consumed in moderation, and some herbalists believe rosemary may even offer postpartum support through mood-lifting and digestive benefits. Monitor the baby for any signs of sensitivity.

Elders (65+)

Rosemary remains a helpful herb in older age — especially for memory, circulation, and mood. However, elders often take medications that rosemary may interact with, such as blood pressure or blood-thinning prescriptions. Starting with smaller doses and monitoring for any shifts in how one feels is a wise approach. Tea and topical preparations are generally well tolerated in moderation.

ROSEMARY NOTES

Personal Experiences

Preparations Tried

Favorite Uses

Blends / Parings

Harvest Notes

Other thoughts

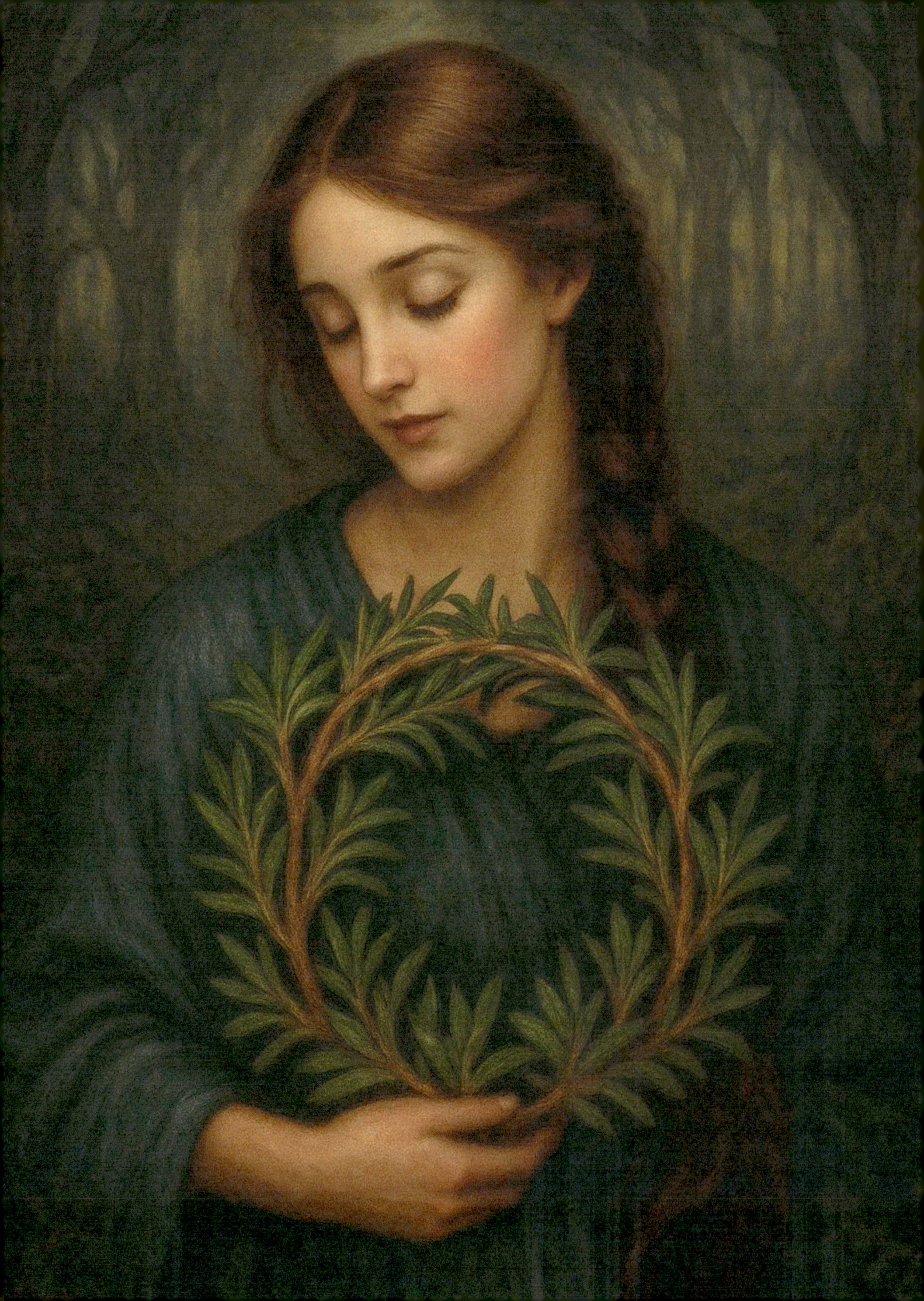

Rosemary: The Herb of Remembrance

Long ago, in the hills of the Mediterranean, rosemary was not yet the fragrant herb we know today. It grew as a humble, green shrub. Useful, yes, but plain. That is, until one sacred night changed everything.

As the story goes, when Mary fled with the infant Jesus into Egypt, she sought shelter along the desert path. Weary and in danger, she stopped beside a rosemary bush. The plant offered her shade from the sun, and its sturdy branches gave her a place to rest.

Needing to wash the baby's clothes, Mary spread them out to dry upon the rosemary's limbs. Grateful for its quiet service, she blessed the plant. From that moment on, the bush was no longer ordinary. It blossomed small blue flowers, the color of Mary's robe, and its leaves took on a sweet, piney fragrance never known before.

From then on, rosemary was called "Rose of Mary." It was said to protect homes from evil, bring healing to the sick, and preserve the memory of those who had passed.

Rosemary whispers

What you protect, will in turn protect you. What you honor, will live on.

THYME

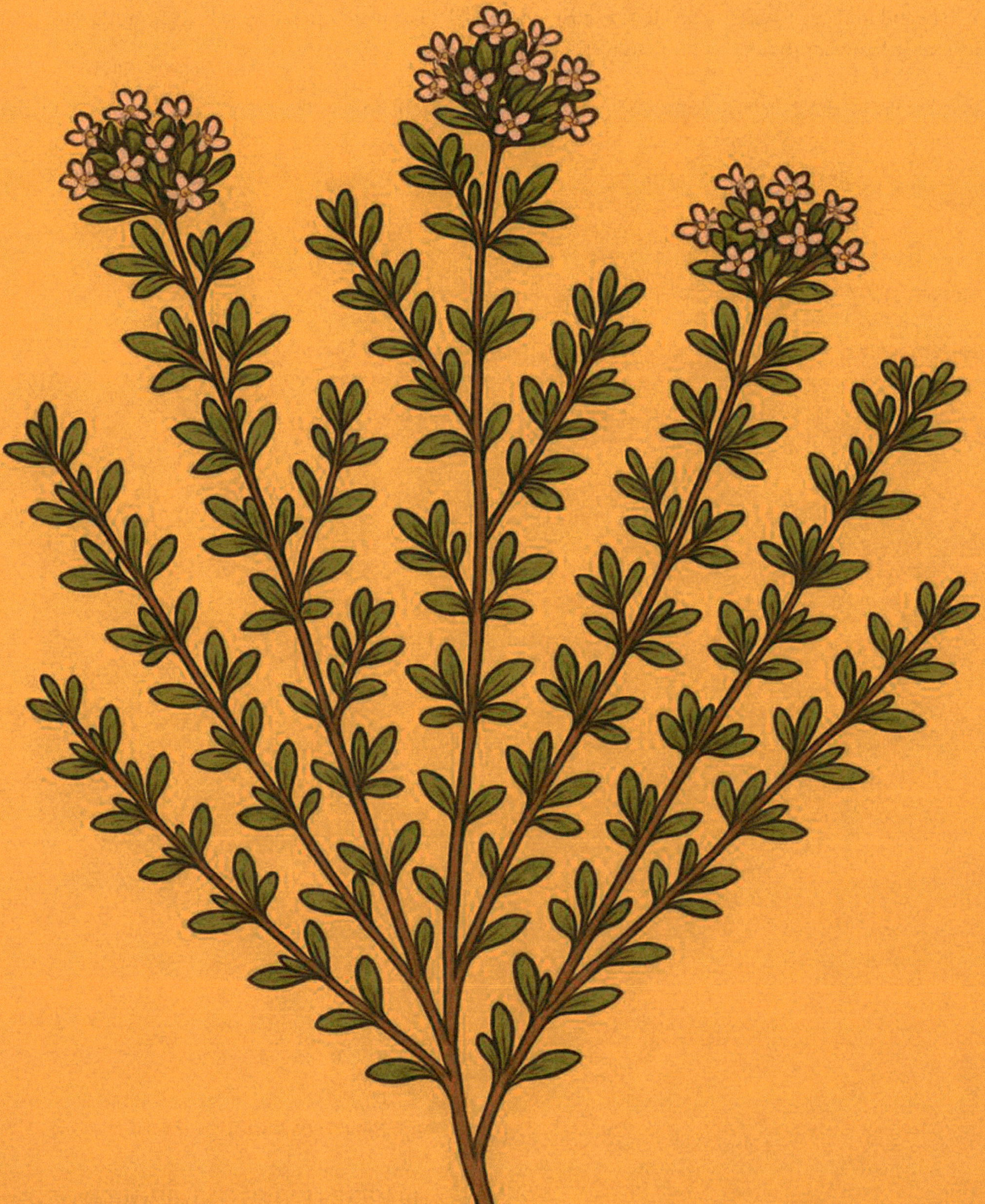

Thyme
(Thymus vulgaris)

Why Grow It?

In summary, it is a must-grow herb for any home garden. Offering both beauty and boldness in a compact, low-maintenance plant, thyme is a staple. Rich in antimicrobial oils, it supports respiratory health, eases digestion, and adds depth to culinary dishes. Its tiny flowers attract pollinators. Whether brewed into tea, infused into oils, or sprinkled on dinner, thyme is versatile, supporting both your kitchen and apothecary needs.

Plant Profile

- **Botanical Name:** Thymus vulgaris
- **Common Names**: Common Thyme, Garden Thyme, Mother of Thyme
- **Family**: Lamiaceae (Mint family)
- **Parts Used:** Leaves and flowering tops
- **Taste:** Pungent, warming, slightly bitter
- **Energetics:** Warming, drying
- **Actions**: Antimicrobial, antispasmodic, carminative, expectorant, immune-stimulating

Botanical Description

Thyme is a low-growing, woody perennial with tiny gray-green leaves and delicate purple or pink flowers. It thrives in dry, sunny locations and is often grown as a culinary and medicinal herb. Its name comes from the Greek thymos, meaning "courage" or "spirit."
Grow Tip: Prefers full sun and well-drained soil. Trim regularly to encourage a bushy shape. Don't over-water.

Medicinal Uses

1. **Respiratory Support**
   - Strong expectorant, helps clear mucus from the lungs.
   - Antimicrobial and antiviral, effective against colds, flu, bronchitis, and sore throats.
   - Used in steam inhalations and teas for congestion, coughs, and sinus infections.

2. **Antimicrobial Powerhouse**
   - Contains thymol, a potent compound that fights bacteria, fungi, and viruses.
   - Useful as a mouthwash, wound wash, or infused oil for topical infections.

3. **Digestive Aid**
    - Stimulates digestion and relieves gas, cramping, and sluggish appetite.
    - Useful in tea or culinary use for food poisoning prevention and gut cleansing.

4. **Nervous System Tonic**
    - Warming and uplifting for mental fatigue, low mood, or fogginess.
    - Promotes courage, clarity, and resilience in times of emotional stress.

Traditional & Folk Uses

- Used by ancient Egyptians in embalming and purification rituals.
- Romans burned thyme to purify air and uplift spirits.
- Placed under pillows in Europe to prevent nightmares.
- Worn or carried as a charm for courage and strength in battle.

Magical & Energetic Associations

- **Element:** Fire
- **Planet:** Venus & Mars
- **Chakra:** Solar Plexus

— Used in spells for courage, protection, purification, and confidence.

— Burned as incense to cleanse spaces and invoke strength.

How to Use Thyme

- **Tea (Infusion):**
  1 tsp dried herb per 8 oz water. Steep 10–15 minutes (covered). Use for colds, flu, digestive support, or general wellness.
- **Tincture:**
  1:5 in 40–50% alcohol. Dose: 20–40 drops as needed.
- **Steam Inhalation:**
  Add a handful of fresh thyme to a bowl of hot water. Inhale deeply for congestion and respiratory relief.
- **Infused Oil / Salve:**
  Used externally for wounds, fungal infections, and muscle aches.
- **Gargle or Mouthwash:**
  Strong infusion cooled and used for sore throats, mouth ulcers, or gum infections.

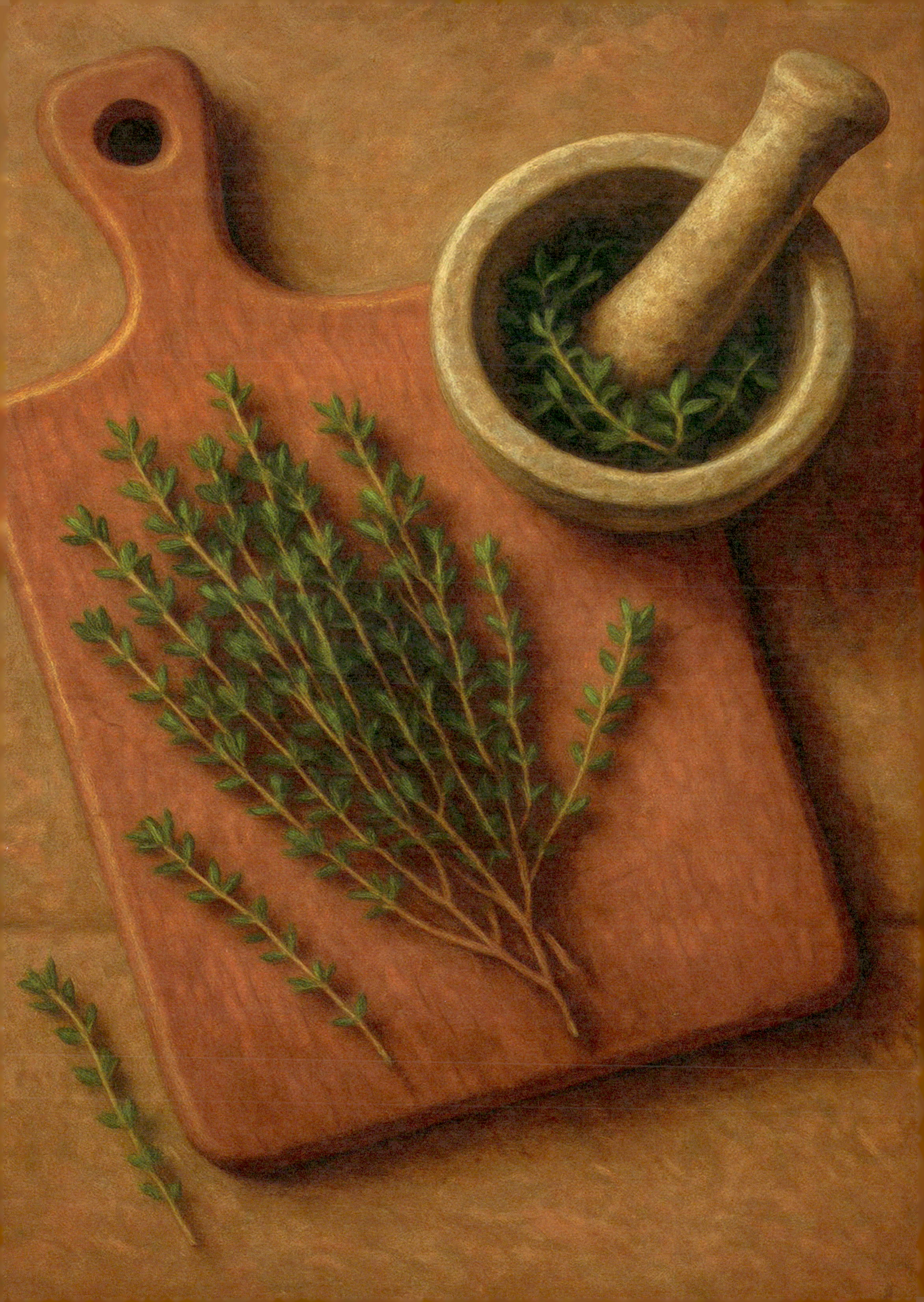

Starting Thyme from Seed

Thyme can be grown from seed, cuttings, or divisions, though it can be slow to germinate.

From Seed

1. Start indoors 6–10 weeks before last frost.
2. Use a light seed-starting mix in trays or small pots.
3. Surface sow or barely cover — thyme seeds need light to germinate.
4. Mist gently to keep soil moist.
5. Germinates in 14–28 days.
6. Transplant when seedlings are 2–3 inches tall.

How to Grow from Cuttings (Easiest Method)

1. Snip a 3–5" stem in spring or summer.
2. Remove lower leaves and place in moist soil or water.
3. Roots form in 2–3 weeks.
4. Transplant into pot or directly into the garden once rooted and stable.

Harvesting Thyme

- Begin harvesting once the plant is 4–6" tall.
- Snip stems just before flowering for the best flavor and aroma.
- Harvest in the morning after dew dries.
- Dry by hanging in bundles or laying flat in a warm, dark space.

Perennial Care

- Hardy in zones 5–9.
- Mulch lightly in winter to protect roots in cold climates.
- Cut back woody growth in early spring to encourage new leaves.
- Replace plants every 4–5 years if they become woody or sparse.

Companion & Pollinator Benefits

- Attracts bees and beneficial insects.
- Deters cabbage moths and whiteflies.
- Excellent companion for brassicas, tomatoes, and eggplants.

Use After Growing

- Infuse in vinegar, honey, or oil.
- Use fresh or dried in tea for coughs, colds, and digestion.
- Burn for cleansing and protection.
- Add to culinary blends, fire cider, or herbal salts.

How to Sprout Thyme from Seed

Supplies

- Thyme seeds
- Seed-starting mix (light, well-draining)
- Seed trays or shallow pots
- Spray bottle or fine watering can
- Clear plastic dome or wrap (optional)
- Sunny windowsill or grow light setup

Step-by-Step Instructions

1. Start indoors 6–10 weeks before your last expected frost.
2. Fill trays with moist seed-starting mix.
3. Surface sow seeds. Thyme seeds are tiny and need light to germinate, so don't bury them — just gently press onto the soil surface.
4. Mist lightly to keep the surface evenly moist (not wet).
5. Cover with a plastic dome or wrap to retain humidity (optional but helpful).
6. Keep warm and bright. Germination temperature: 65–75°F (18–24°C).
7. Be patient — thyme seeds take 14–28 days to germinate (sometimes longer in cooler temps).
8. Remove cover and thin seedlings once true leaves appear.
9. Transplant when seedlings are about 2–3 inches tall and after hardening off.

After Sprouting

- Plant in full sun, 12–18 inches apart.
- Water deeply but let soil dry out between waterings.
- Avoid overwatering — thyme thrives in lean, dry soil.

Can You Eat Thyme Sprouts?

Technically yes, but:

- They're tiny, slow-growing, and a bit woody even when young.
- Not used as microgreens.
- Thyme's flavor and medicinal potency are best when fully grown and dried or used fresh.

Thyme Herbal Tea Sipping Chart

Form	Amount per 8oz water	Seeping Time	Best for
Fresh	2–3 tsp lightly bruised	10–12 minutes	Sore throat, immune support, clarity
Dried	1 tsp crushed	8–10 minutes	Chest colds, coughs, digestion, focus
Strong Infusion	1 Tbsp dried	15+ minutes	Respiratory relief, sinus steam
Cold brew	2 Tbsp dried or fresh	4–6 hours (fridge)	Cooling digestive aid, antioxidant sip

Benefits of Thyme Tea

- Soothes gut lining (ulcers, leaky gut, reflux)
- Moves lymph and clears skin from the inside out
- Eases inflammation and supports healing
- Gentle antimicrobial and antifungal action

Safety of Thyme by Age Group

Infants (Under 1 Year)

Not recommended.

Thyme contains potent essential oils (like thymol) that can be too strong for an infant's developing system.

Children (1–6 years)

- Use low-dose preparations only: ¼ teaspoon dried herb per 8 oz cup, steeped briefly (5 min), and offered in small amounts (2–4 oz max/day).
- Ideal in diluted blends for coughs or colds but best under guidance if used frequently.

Children (7–12 years)

- Can tolerate ½–1 cup of weak tea per day, made with ½–1 tsp dried thyme.
- Monitor for sensitivity or tummy upset.
- Great for respiratory support and mild digestive issues.

Teens & Adults

- Generally safe and well-tolerated in culinary or tea doses: 1–3 cups/day using 1 tsp dried thyme per 8 oz.
- Avoid excessive intake or concentrated tinctures long-term due to potential thyroid effects.

Pregnancy & Breastfeeding

- Moderate use in food and tea is considered safe.
- Avoid highly concentrated forms (e.g., thyme essential oil or strong decoctions).
- Helpful for digestion and immunity in late pregnancy—check with a midwife or herbalist.

Elderly

- Often very beneficial for aging lungs, weak digestion, and immune support.
- Monitor with blood pressure medications, anticoagulants, or thyroid medications—thyme may mildly interact in large doses.
- One of the gentler respiratory allies when used in normal tea strength.

THYME NOTES

Personal Experiences

Preparations Tried

Favorite Uses

Blends / Parings

Harvest Notes

Other thoughts

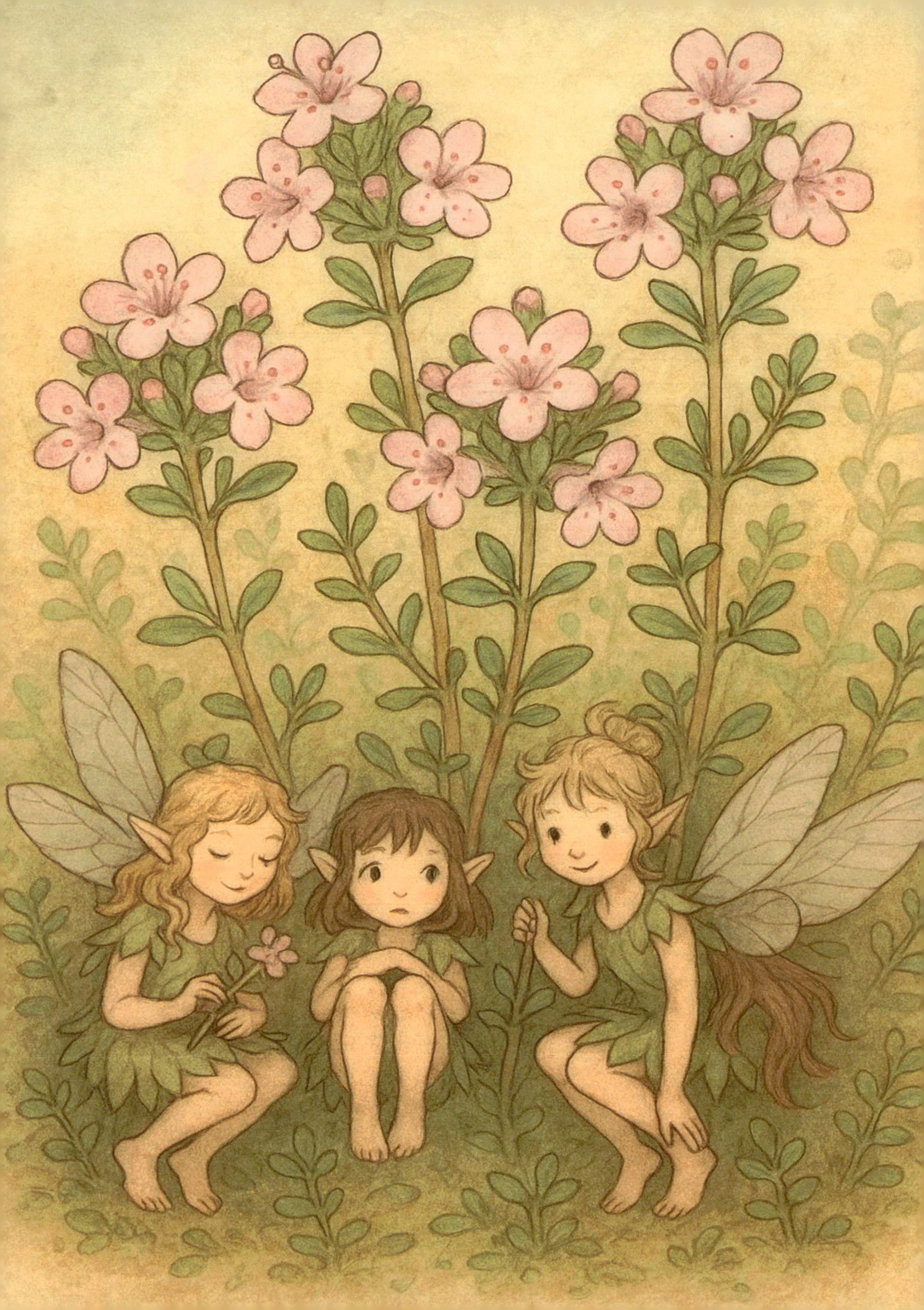

Thyme: The Herb of Courage and the Fairy Veil

In a misty village nestled at the edge of the woods, there lived an old herbalist known only as Nanna Thyra. Children whispered that she talked to plants, and some swore they saw flickers of light dancing in her herb garden after dusk.

One day, a frightened young boy came to her door. He was small and quiet, often bullied by others, and too afraid to speak up for himself. "I wish I were brave," he told her. "Like the stories. Like the knights, the foxes, and the fire."

Nanna Thyra smiled, reached into her garden, and plucked a sprig of a low-growing herb with tiny purple flowers. "This," she said, "is thyme. It's not loud. It doesn't shout. But it will help you remember who you are."

She brewed him a tea, then showed him how to rub the leaves between his fingers to release their scent. "Thyme is for courage, boy. Even the smallest warrior needs it."

That night, he placed the thyme under his pillow and dreamed of a circle of fairies, dancing in a glade filled with moonlight. One whispered, "He who carries thyme may see us, and he who drinks it may find his voice."

From that day forward, the boy walked a little taller. He still wasn't loud—but he spoke with clarity, and the others listened. And some say, on Midsummer's Eve, he returned to the fairy glade and was granted a charm: a sprig of thyme that never wilted.

Thyme in Folk Magic and Lore

- Burned in homes to ward off sorrow, bad dreams, and illness.
- Used in baths or teas to give courage before battle or challenge.
- Believed to allow humans to see fairies if gathered at dawn on Midsummer.
- Slipped into pillows to inspire restful dreams and bravery in sleep.
- Associated with love, strength, purification, and ancestral memory.

Thyme Teaches

Quiet courage is still courage. Even the smallest leaf can guard a heart, stir the soul, and open the unseen.

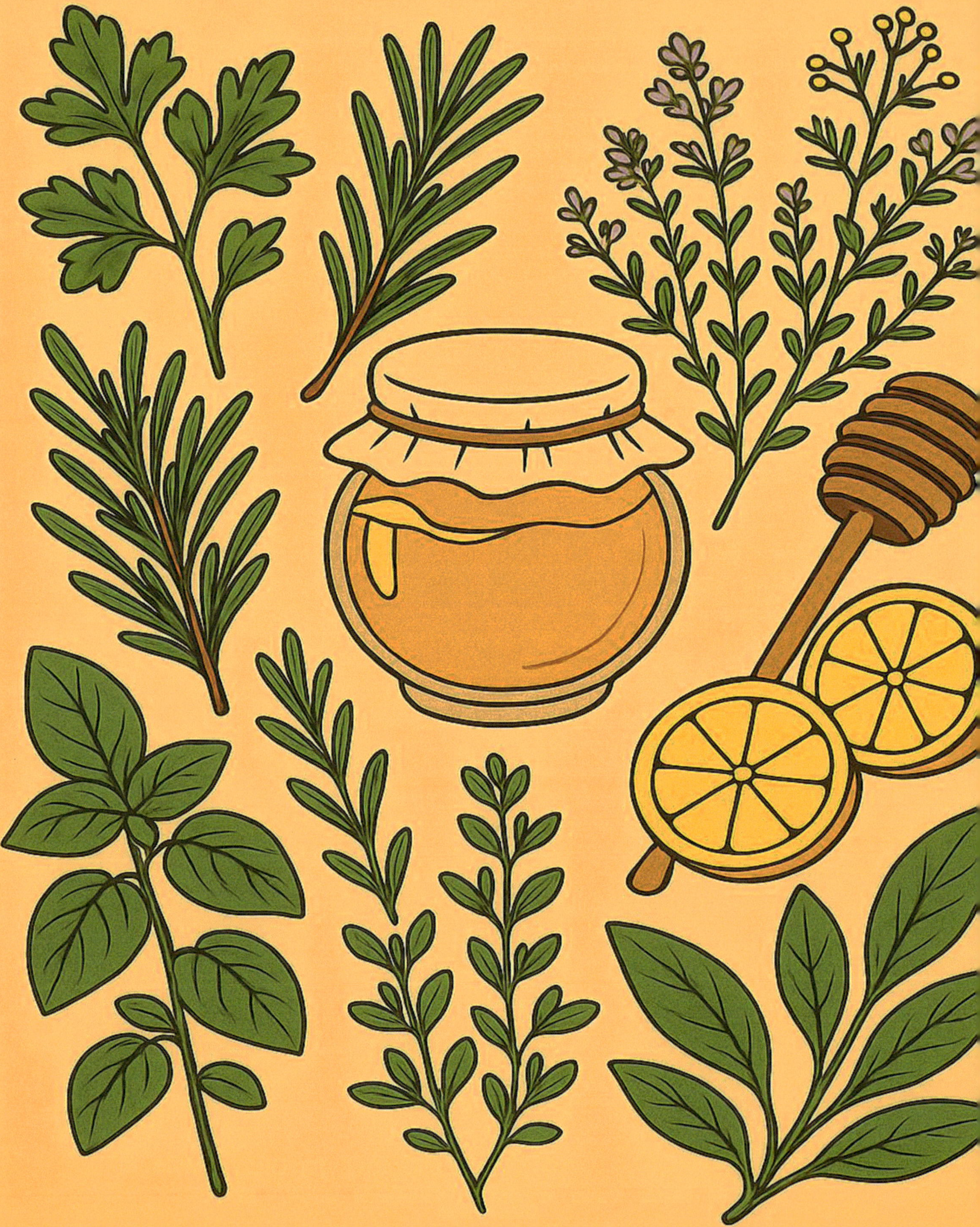

Over 100 Recipes: 3 Ingredients or Less, Using the 10 Herbs Everyone Should Grow

Quick Reference: This section is designed for the seasoned naturalist who doesn't need step-by-step instructions. Just simple ingredients, blends, and combinations. Once you've mastered your technique, this list will provide you with a quick reference. Be sure to utilize the **Notes** section at the end of each chapter. It's a great way to remember what you've tried and what worked. Under each heading is a page reference for the step-by-step instructions.

Herbal Tea Blends (serve with local honey, lemon wedge, or zest)

1 Tbsp herb to 8oz water

1. **Lemon Balm Calming Tea** – lemon balm + honey + hot water
2. **Sleepy Chamomile Tea** – chamomile + lavender + hot water
3. **Digestive Peppermint Tea** – peppermint + lemon balm + hot water
4. **Digestion Soothe, Emotional Balance & Circulatory Support** – chamomile + holy basil + hot water
5. **Holy Basil Adaptogen Brew** – holy basil + ginger + hot water
6. **Detox Nettle Tea** – nettle + lemon slice + hot water
7. **Thyme Cold Support Tea** – thyme + honey + hot water
8. **Rosemary Brain Boost Tea** – rosemary + orange peel + hot water
9. **Calendula Glow Tea** – calendula + lemon balm + nettle + hot water
10. **Calendula Sunshine** – calendula + lemon balm + peppermint + hot water
11. **Uplift & Energy** – lemon balm + rosemary + peppermint
12. **Morning Clarity** – rosemary + lemon balm + honey
13. **Heart & Harmony** – holy basil + lemon balm + chamomile
14. **Lavender Relaxation Tea** – lavender + chamomile + hot water
15. **Allergy Ease** – nettle + chamomile + holy basil + hot water
16. **Nourish & Restore** – nettle, holy basil, peppermint
17. **Seasonal Shield** – rosemary + sage + thyme + peppermint
18. **Breath of Wild Air** – thyme + peppermint + nettle + hot water
19. **Breathe & Balance** – thyme + sage + holy basil
20. **Berry Herb Cooler** – lemon balm + peppermint + hot water (serve iced with honey, berries, and lemon)
21. **Sage Sore Throat Tea** – sage + sea salt + hot water (for gargling)
22. **Minty Fresh Breath Gargle** – peppermint + thyme + sea salt + hot water (for gargling)
23. **Garden Gratitude Tea** – a pinch of whatever speaks to you, measure with your heart

Herbal Drinks & Tonics

24. **Peppermint Lime Cooler** – peppermint + lime + sparkling water
25. **Nettle Tonic Vinegar** – nettle + apple cider vinegar
26. **Holy Basil Iced Tea** – holy basil + honey + ice
27. **Herbal Tonic** – holy basil + rosemary + ½ lemon + 12 oz water
28. **Lemon Balm Sparkle** – lemon balm + ½ lemon + sparkling water
29. **Calendula Citrus Cooler** – calendula + peppermint + orange peel + honey

Herb-Infused Honeys

1 cup raw local honey + ¼–½ cup dried herb of choice (or ½–1 cup fresh)

30. **Calming Tea Sweetener** – lemon balm + raw honey
31. **Thyme Infused Honey** – thyme + honey
32. **Calendula Sunshine Honey** – calendula petals + honey
33. **Chamomile Sleep Honey** – chamomile + honey
34. **Calming Bedtime Sweetener Honey** – chamomile + lemon balm + honey
35. **For Sore Throats & Winter Wellness** – thyme + sage + honey
36. **Stress Reducing** – holy basil + honey
37. **Balancing & Antimicrobial** – sage + honey
38. **Uplifting and Aromatic** – lavender + mint + honey
39. **Gentle Skin-Supporting Blend** – calendula + honey
40. **Digestive Relief** – peppermint + honey
41. **Rosemary + Peppermint + Honey**

Culinary Herbal Salts

1 part herb to 4 parts salt or 1 Tbsp herb to ½ cup salt

42. **Rosemary Salt** – dried rosemary + sea salt
43. **Healing Broth Salt** – nettle + rosemary + sage + sea salt
44. **Fruit Salad Salt** – peppermint + lemon balm + sea salt
45. **Vegetable Salt** – rosemary + thyme + sage + sea salt
46. **Sage Garlic Salt** – sage + garlic powder + sea salt
47. **Thyme Lemon Zest Salt** – thyme + lemon zest + sea salt
48. **Lemon Herb Salt** – rosemary + sage + lemon zest + sea salt
49. **Lemon Balm Citrus Salt** – lemon balm + lemon zest + sea salt

Culinary Herb Butters

1 stick unsalted butter to 1-2 Tbsp fresh herb (tsp dried)

50. **Sage Butter** – sage + unsalted butter
51. **Calendula Butter Spread** – calendula + butter
52. **Butter for Bread, Potatoes, or Roasting** – garlic + parsley + thyme + unsalted butter
53. **Butter for Muffins, Scones, or Toast** – lemon balm + honey + unsalted butter
54. **Butter for Grilled Meats** – rosemary + sage + sea salt + unsalted butter

Culinary Infused Olive Oils

¼–½ cup dried herbs + 1 cup quality olive oil

55. **Thyme-Infused Olive Oil** – thyme + olive oil
56. **Rosemary Infused Olive Oil** – rosemary + olive oil (delicious on potatoes)
57. **Calendula & Holy Basil Infused Olive Oil** – calendula + holy basil + olive oil (adds a golden color and calm energy to salads and soups)
58. **Lemon Balm & Sage Infused Olive Oil** – great on fish, chicken, & summer squash

Topical Remedies

59. **Calendula Salve** – calendula-infused oil + beeswax
60. **Chamomile Infused Oil** – for calming skin, facial or salve base
61. **Calendula Infused Oil** – for calming skin, facial or salve base
62. **Rosemary Infused Oil** – great for hair growth and circulation
63. **Thyme or Sage Oil** – use in salves for sore muscles or chest rubs
64. **Lemon Balm Infused Oil** – for stress relief and bedtime blends
65. **Sage or Rosemary Infused Oil** – for scalp massage or sore muscles
66. **Holy Basil or Nettle Infused Oil** – for energizing, antioxidant-rich oils
67. **Peppermint + Thyme Infused Oil** – for freshening foot oil or chest rub
68. **Sage Vinegar Rinse** – sage + apple cider vinegar

Simple DIY Bath & Body

69. **Lavender Bath Soak** – lavender + Epsom salts
70. **Chamomile Oat Bath** – chamomile + oats
71. **Rosemary Foot Soak** – rosemary + Epsom salts
72. **Thyme Steam Bowl** – thyme + hot water (for congestion)
73. **Chamomile + Lemon Balm + Calendula Steam Bowl** – for glow & calm skin
74. **Rosemary + Thyme + Sage + Peppermint Steam Bowl** – for respiratory support

75. **Holy Basil + Lemon Balm + Nettle Steam Bowl** – for the nervous system
76. **Rosemary + Thyme + Sage Steam Bowl** – for sinus support
77. **Peppermint Sugar Scrub** – peppermint + sugar + coconut oil
78. **Relaxing Bedtime Sugar Scrub** – lavender + chamomile + sugar
79. **Energizing Morning Sugar Scrub** – mint + rosemary + sugar
80. **Brightening and Soothing Sugar Scrub** – calendula + sugar + lemon zest (optional)
81. **Nettle Vinegar Hair Rinse** – nettle + apple cider vinegar
82. **Strength Hair Rinse** – rosemary + nettle + calendula + water
83. **Herbal Bath** – chamomile + calendula
84. **Herbal Bath** – Epsom salt + rosemary + holy basil
85. **Chamomile Hand Balm** – 2 parts chamomile-infused oil + 1 part beeswax
86. **Cooling Foot Spray** – 1 Tbsp peppermint + 1 Tbsp witch hazel + 1 cup water

Treats & Snacks

87. **Shortbread Bites** – herb + butter + flour (see pg for more ideas and instructions)
88. **Peppermint Chocolate Bark** – peppermint + dark chocolate
89. **Calendula Jelly** – calendula tea + sugar + pectin
90. **Thyme Popcorn** – thyme + oil + popcorn
91. **Sage Crackers** – sage + flour + water
92. **Rosemary Crackers** – rosemary + flour + water
93. **Holy Basil Crackers** – holy basil + parmesan + flour + water
94. **Sage Crackers** – sage + onion powder + flour + water

Home Uses

95. **Chamomile Pillow Sachets** – chamomile + cotton bag
96. **Lavender Drawer Freshener** – lavender + rice (in sachet)
97. **Simmer Pots** – (see pg for more ideas and instructions)
98. **Sage Smoke Cleanse Bundle** – dried sage + string
99. **Lemon Balm Room Spray** – lemon balm tea + vodka + water
100. **Relax Room Spray** – lavender + chamomile, sage + vodka + water
101. **Focus Room Spray** – rosemary + peppermint + vodka + water
102. **Cleanse Room Spray** – sage + vodka + water

NOTES

Personal Experiences

Preparations Tried

Favorite Uses

Blends / Parings

Harvest Notes

Other thoughts

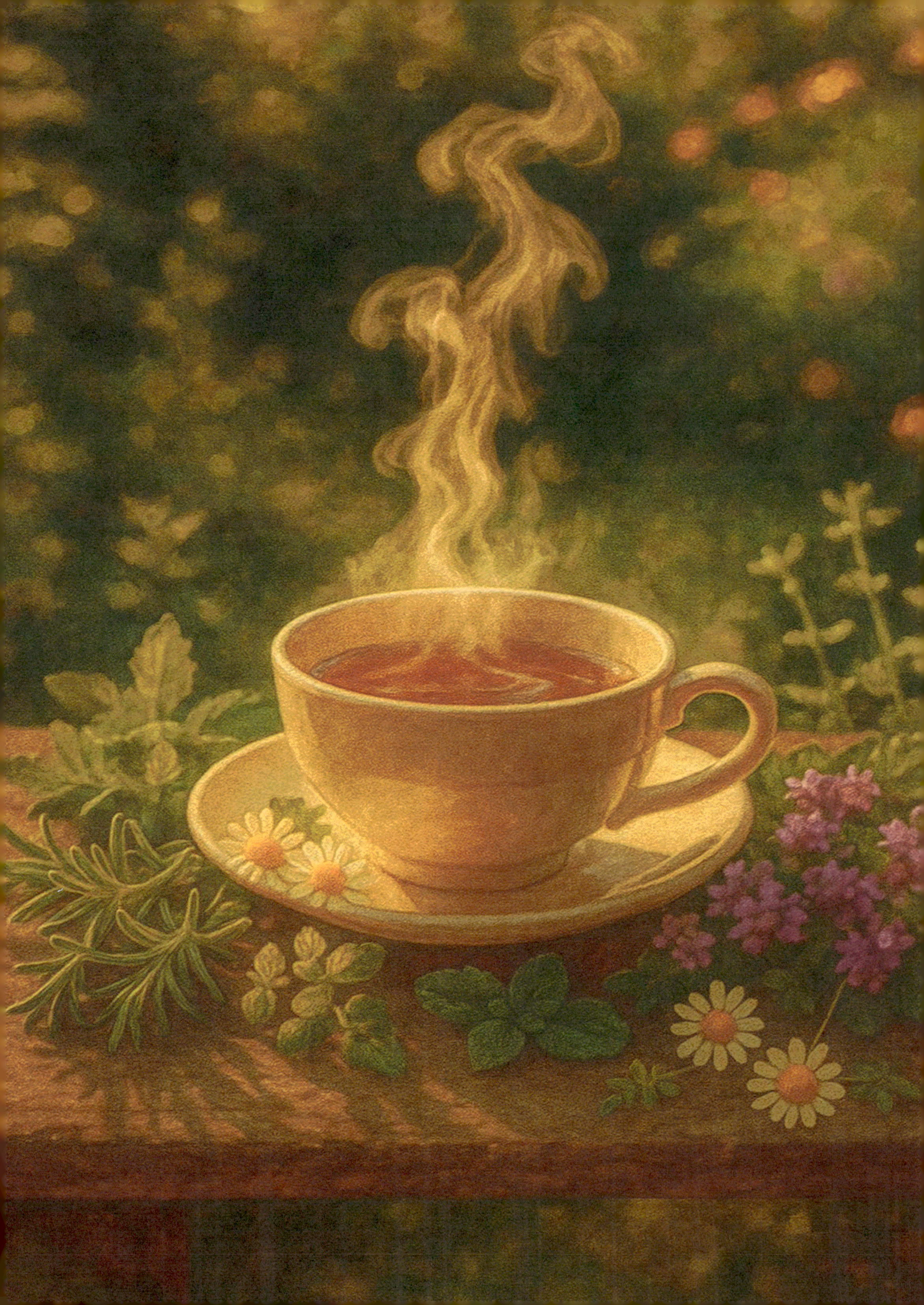

Tea: A Connection to Nature and Tradition

Some people have a coffee station. I have a tea station. No pods. No frother. Just jars of my top 10 herbal staples and a jar of my favorite local honey. Each one grown with care, harvested in season, and ready to soothe, energize, or simply bring comfort in a warm mug. Because tea isn't just a drink, it's a daily way to connect with nature, with tradition, and with yourself.

What Is a Tea?

An herbal tea is simply an infusion of plants in hot water. Unlike black or green teas (which come from the Camellia sinensis plant), herbal teas use leaves, flowers, seeds, roots, or stems from other healing plants to extract flavor and benefits.

Teas are one of the easiest and most traditional ways to enjoy the gentle power of herbs. With just a few minutes of steeping, a cup of tea can offer comfort, support, and nourishment.

Why Start with Tea?

Tea is one of the simplest, most accessible ways to begin this journey. True healing doesn't come from masking the symptoms. It begins deep within, where the body, mind, and spirit find space to restore themselves. Herbal tea is real nourishment.

How to Brew Herbal Tea - Basic Herbal Tea (Infusion)

Best for: Leaves & flowers (like lemon balm, calendula, or mint)

1. **Boil Water**: Use fresh, clean water and bring it just to a boil.
2. **Measure Herbs**: Use 1 teaspoon of dried herb or 1 tablespoon of fresh herb per cup of water.
3. **Steep Covered**: Pour hot water over herbs, cover the cup or teapot, and steep for 5–15 minutes.
4. **Strain & Sip**: Remove herbs, add honey or lemon if desired, and enjoy warm or chilled.

Stronger Infusions (Medicinal Use)

Steep longer (up to 1–4 hours) for a more potent brew, especially when using herbs for deeper wellness support.

Decoctions (For Roots & Barks)

Best for: Tougher parts like roots or seeds (like nettle root or cinnamon bark)

1. **Add to Cold Water**: Place herbs in a pot with cold water.
2. **Simmer Gently**: Bring to a gentle boil, then simmer for 15–30 minutes.
3. **Strain & Enjoy**: Let cool slightly, strain, and serve.

Sip it Sweet ~ Honey

Why Use Organic, Local Honey in Your Herbal Teas?

Not all honey is created equal. When crafting herbal teas that support wellness, the quality of your honey matters just as much as the herbs you grow. Here's why you should reach for organic, local honey when sweetening your brews:

1. **It Preserves the Purpose of the Tea**
   Herbal teas are often brewed for specific intentions: to soothe, restore, energize, or calm. Using raw, local honey ensures you're adding a natural, living ingredient that supports, rather than disrupts those intentions.
   - Commercial honey is often pasteurized or cut with syrups. These syrups strip away its natural enzymes and healing benefits.
   - Organic, raw honey contains beneficial enzymes, antioxidants, and trace nutrients that complement herbal actions.
2. **It Connects You to the Land and the Bees**
   Just as your herbs are rooted in the soil around you, local honey reflects the flowers, trees, and terrain of your region. It's a beautiful act of reciprocity: the bees pollinate your herbs, and you use their gift in your brews.
   - Local honey can gently support seasonal allergy relief, as it contains micro-traces of local pollen.
   - Supporting local beekeepers helps preserve healthy bee populations, which are essential for your garden and the planet.
3. **It Avoids Hidden Chemicals and Contaminants**
   Mass-market honey can contain pesticide residues, antibiotics, or be sourced from unknown international suppliers. Even "organic" honey sold nationally may not meet the same standards as your neighborhood beekeeper's harvest.
   - Local, small-batch honey is more likely to be harvested with care, free of additives or ultra-filtration.
4. **It Honors the Integrity of Your Practice**
   Herbal tea is more than just a drink, it's a ritual, a medicine, a story. Choosing honey that's ethical, intentional, and local aligns with the spirit of what you're creating.
   - When you blend herbs from your garden and sweeten them with honey from nearby hives, you create a cup of tea that is wildly, wonderfully yours.

Final Tip: Always add honey after your tea has cooled slightly; very hot water can destroy the beneficial enzymes in raw honey. Aim for under 110°F when stirring it in.

TEA NOTES

Personal Experiences

Preparations Tried

Favorite Uses

Blends / Parings

Harvest Notes

Other thoughts

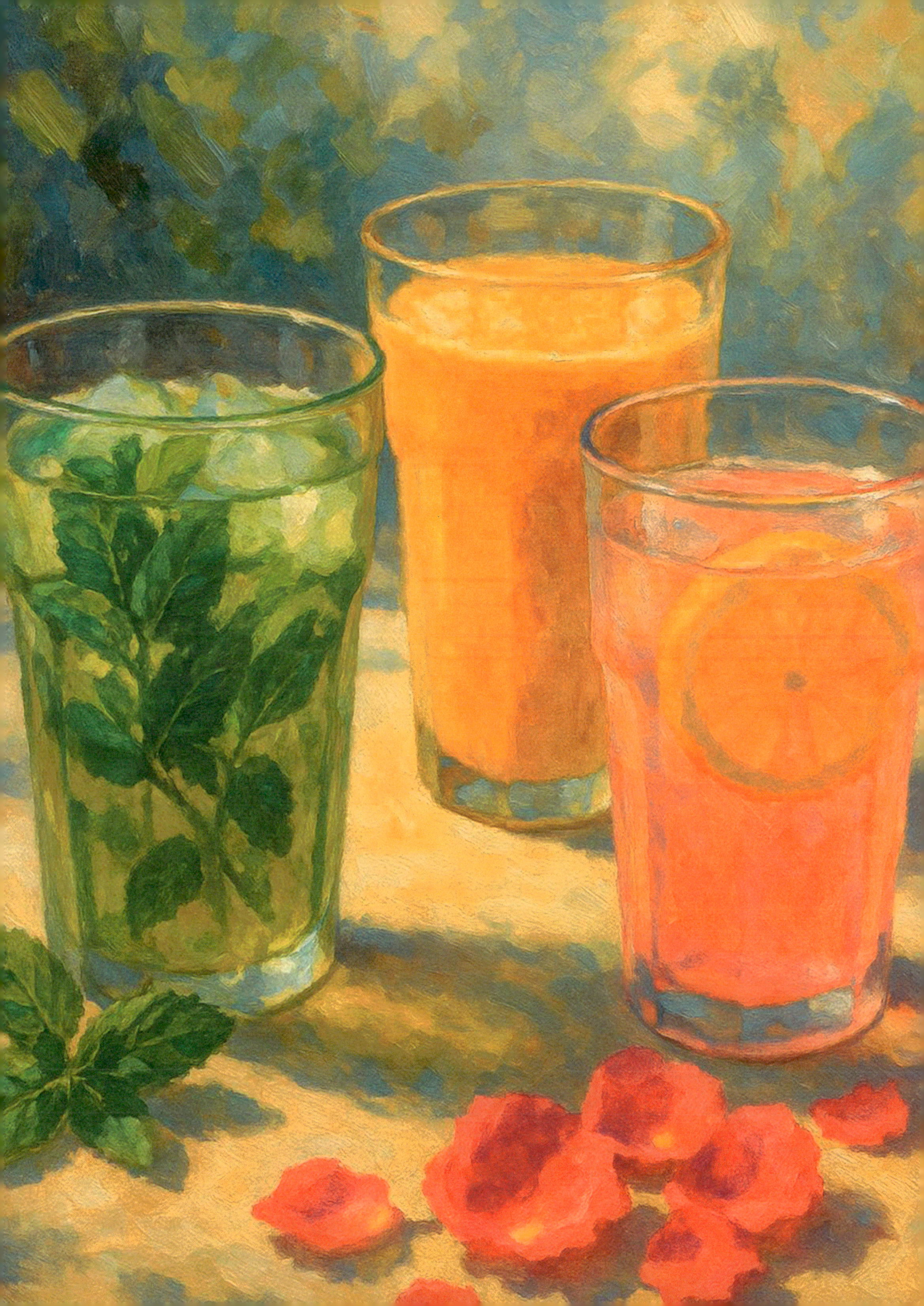

Herbal Drinks & Tonics Using the 10 Herbs Everyone Should Grow

Herbal drinks are more than just teas. They're cooling infusions, sparkling mocktails, and sipping vinegars. Wellness tonics support your body, calm your mind, and celebrate the beauty of your homegrown herbs. Each of the drinks below can be made with fresh or dried herbs and sweetened to taste with local honey, maple syrup, or fruit juice.

Lemon Balm Sparkle

Uplifting + mood-brightening

• 1 handful fresh lemon balm
• Juice of ½ lemon
• Sparkling water
• Optional: splash of honey or elderflower syrup

Steep lemon balm in hot water for 10 minutes, cool, strain, and mix with sparkling water and lemon. Pour over ice.

Calendula Citrus Cooler

Skin-supportive + cooling

• 1 tbsp dried calendula petals
• 1 tsp dried peppermint
• 1 orange peel strip
• Honey or agave (optional)

Steep herbs and peel in 1–2 cups hot water. Let cool and serve over ice with a slice of orange.

Holy Basil Morning Tonic

Adaptogenic + energizing without caffeine

• 1 tbsp dried holy basil (Tulsi)
• 1 tsp dried lemon balm
• 1 tsp dried rosemary
• Dash of raw apple cider vinegar

Steep herbs for 10–15 minutes. Strain, cool, and add 1–2 tsp ACV and a drizzle of honey. Drink first thing in the morning for clarity and energy.

Mint + Nettle Mineral Iced Tea

Replenishing + deeply nourishing

- 1 tbsp dried nettle
- 1 tbsp fresh or dried peppermint
- 2 cups boiling water

Steep for 30 minutes to 4 hours (longer = stronger mineral draw). Chill and serve over ice with cucumber or lemon.

Thyme & Sage Digestive Tonic

Warming + gut-supportive
- 1 tsp dried thyme
- 1 tsp dried sage
- 1 tbsp apple cider vinegar
- ½ tsp raw honey

Steep herbs, let cool, then mix with vinegar and honey. Drink 1–2 tbsp diluted in water before meals.

Herbal Shrub (Sipping Vinegar)

Sweet + tangy summer tonic

Use any combo of -
- Peppermint, rosemary, or lemon balm
- Fruit (like berries, peaches, or citrus)
- Raw apple cider vinegar
- Honey or maple syrup

Let steep in the fridge for 3–5 days. Strain and serve mixed with sparkling water.

TONIC NOTES

Personal Experiences

Preparations Tried

Favorite Uses

Blends / Parings

Harvest Notes

Other thoughts

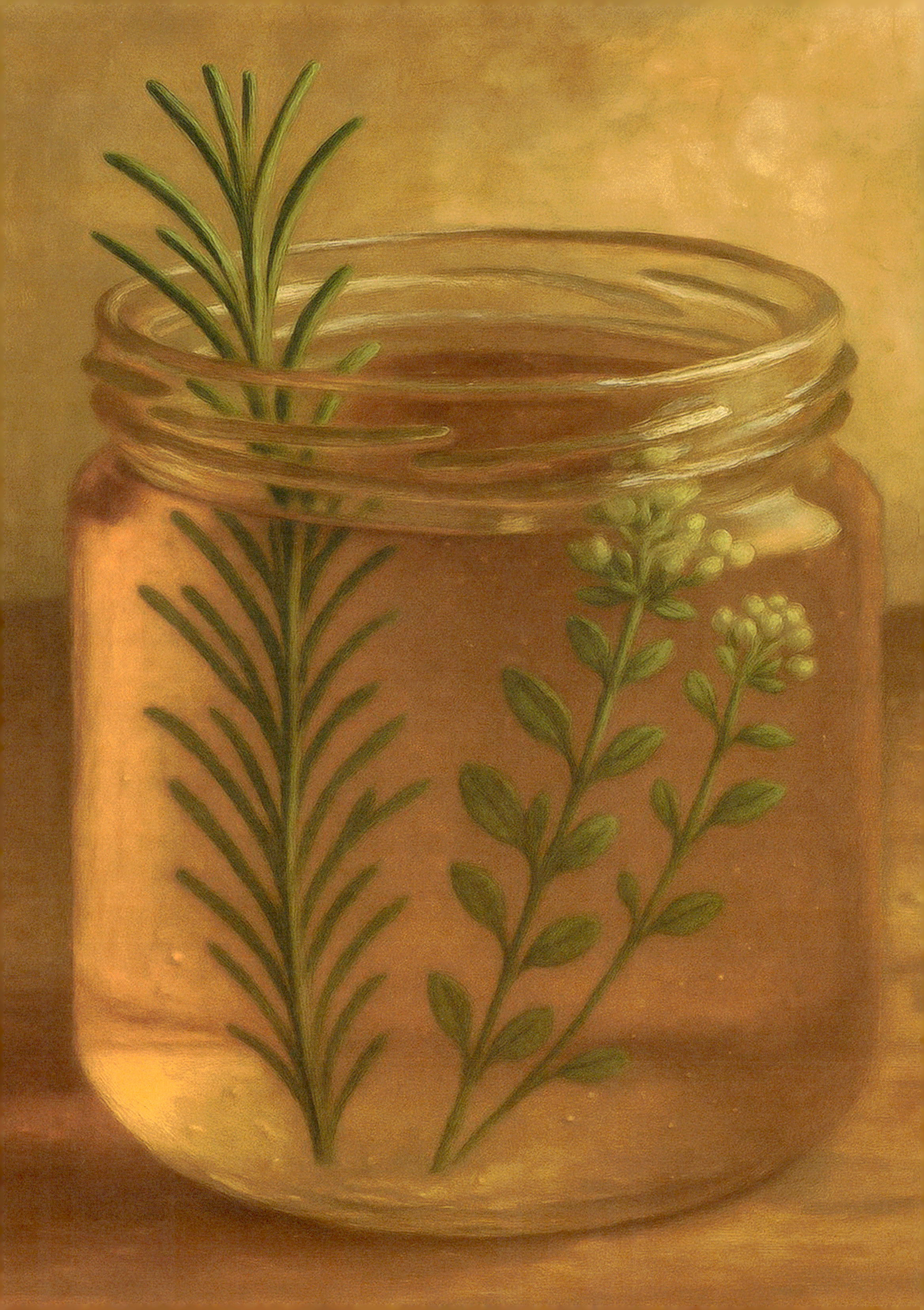

HERBAL-INFUSED HONEY

Here's a simple set of instructions for making herb-infused honey (perfect for teas, toast, or remedies). This version works beautifully with any of your 10 core herbs.

Ingredients

- 1 cup raw local honey
- ¼–½ cup dried herb of choice (or ½–1 cup fresh)

Instructions

Prepare Your Herbs:

- If using fresh herbs, allow them to wilt for 12–24 hours to reduce moisture (this helps prevent spoilage).
- Lightly crush dried herbs with your hands or a mortar and pestle to release oils.

Combine Honey & Herbs:

- Place the herbs into a clean, dry glass jar. Pour honey over them slowly, using a spoon or skewer to release air bubbles and ensure all herbs are submerged.

Infuse Naturally (No-Heat Method):

- Cap the jar and let it sit in a sunny windowsill or warm spot for 1–2 weeks, turning the jar daily to keep herbs evenly coated.

Optional: For quicker results, gently warm the honey jar in a warm water bath (below 100°F) for a few hours.

Strain (Optional):

- After infusing, you may strain out the herbs with a fine mesh sieve or cheesecloth—or leave them in for a rustic touch.

Store & Enjoy:

- Keep in a cool, dark place. Infused honey is shelf-stable and will last for months. Always use clean utensils to avoid contamination.

INFUSED HONEY NOTES

Personal Experiences

Preparations Tried

Favorite Uses

Blends / Parings

Harvest Notes

Other thoughts

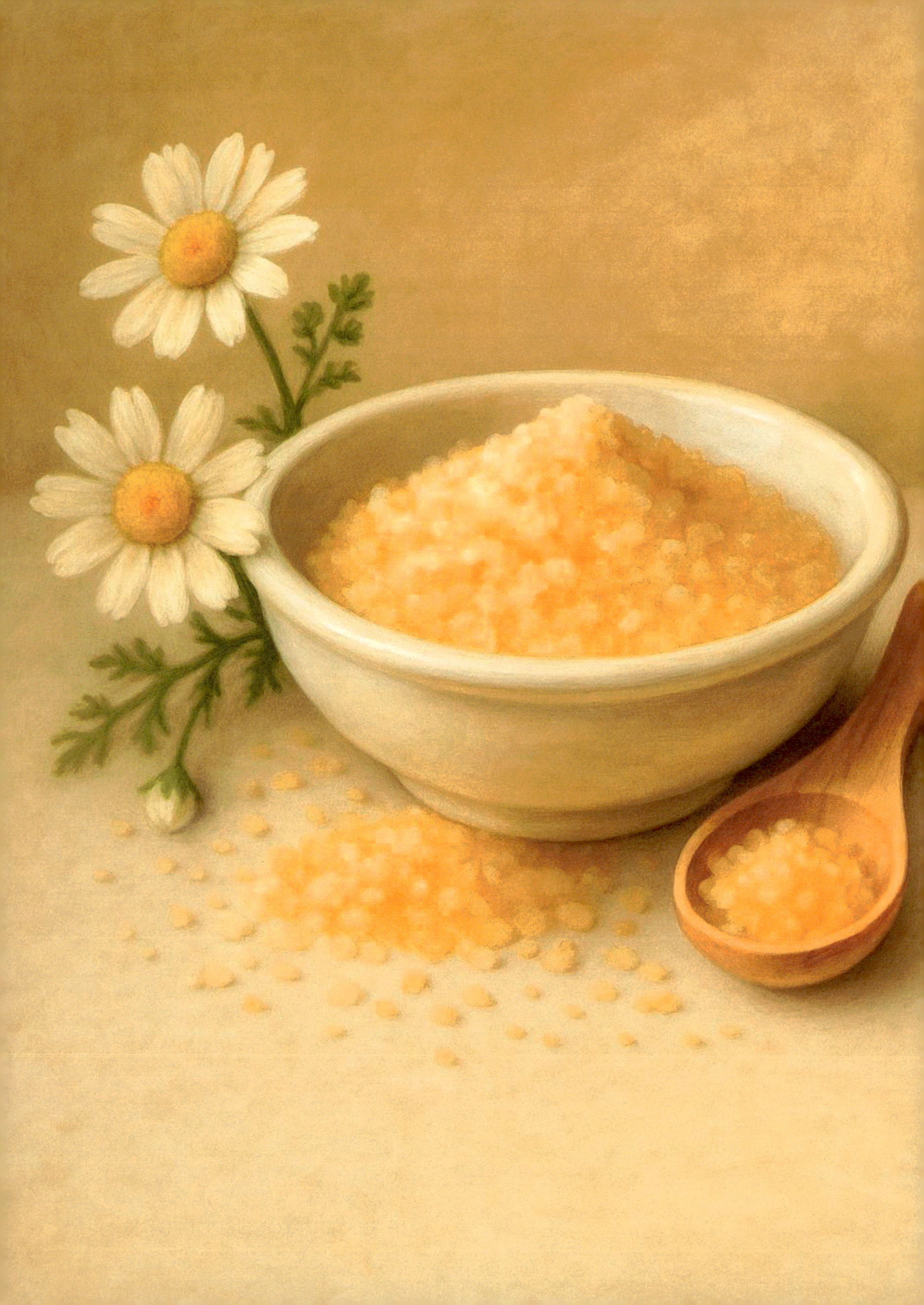

What Are Culinary Herbal Salts?

Herbal salts are flavorful blends made by combining culinary herbs with natural salts. They pair well with vegetables and offer a simple way to bring both flavor and function to everyday meals. Along with trace minerals, they aid digestion and offer gentle wellness support.

They're easy to make, store beautifully, and are a great way to preserve garden herbs or wild harvests. Use them to season roasted veggies, sprinkle on salads, rim a cocktail glass, or gift in tiny jars.

How to Make Herbal Salt

You'll Need:

- Dried herbs of your choice (like rosemary, thyme, sage, basil)
- Natural salt (coarse sea salt, kosher salt, or Himalayan pink)

Instructions:

1. **Choose Your Ratio:**
   Start with about 1 part herbs to 4 parts salt—adjust to taste.
2. **Grind or Mix:**
   Use a mortar & pestle or food processor to blend herbs and salt. For a rustic look, simply mix without grinding.
3. **Dry If Needed:**
   Spread on a baking sheet and let air dry (or gently heat in the oven on low, 150°F or below, for 10–15 minutes) to prevent clumping.
4. **Store:**
   Transfer to a clean glass jar with a label and keep in a cool, dry spot.

CULINARY HERB SALT NOTES

Personal Experiences

Preparations Tried

Favorite Uses

Blends / Parings

Harvest Notes

Other thoughts

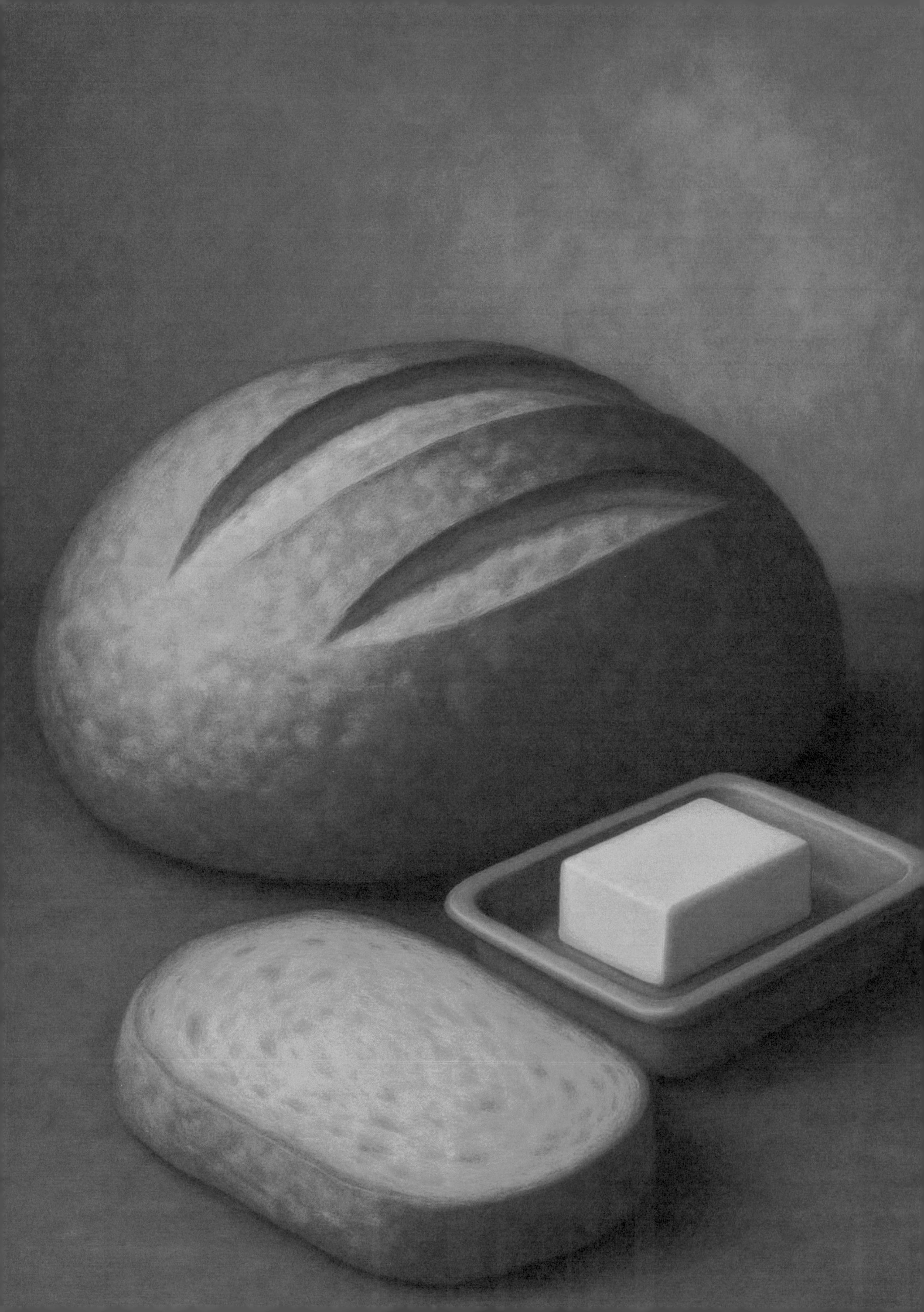

What Is Herb Butter?

Herb butter is a flavorful blend of softened butter mixed with fresh or dried herbs, spices, citrus zest, or even edible flowers. It's a simple and delicious way to preserve seasonal herbs and bring gourmet flavor to everyday meals.

Sometimes called compound butter, it's perfect for spreading on bread, melting over vegetables or grilled meats, stirring into pasta, or using in baking. Herb butters can be savory or sweet. They are easy to make ahead and freeze for later use.

How to Make Herb Butter

You'll Need

- ½ cup (1 stick) unsalted butter, softened
- 1–2 tablespoons finely chopped fresh herbs (or 1 tsp dried)
- Optional: garlic, lemon zest, edible flowers, salt, honey, or spices

Instructions

1. **Soften the Butter:**
   Leave at room temperature until easily spreadable.
2. **Mix It Up:**
   In a bowl, stir together butter, herbs, and any extras.
3. **Shape & Store:**
   Spoon onto parchment paper and roll into a log, or press into a small jar or dish. Chill until firm.

Tip: Wrap in parchment and label for gifting, or freeze in slices to add instant flavor to meals.

CULINARY HERB BUTTER NOTES

Personal Experiences

Preparations Tried

Favorite Uses

Blends / Parings

Harvest Notes

Other thoughts

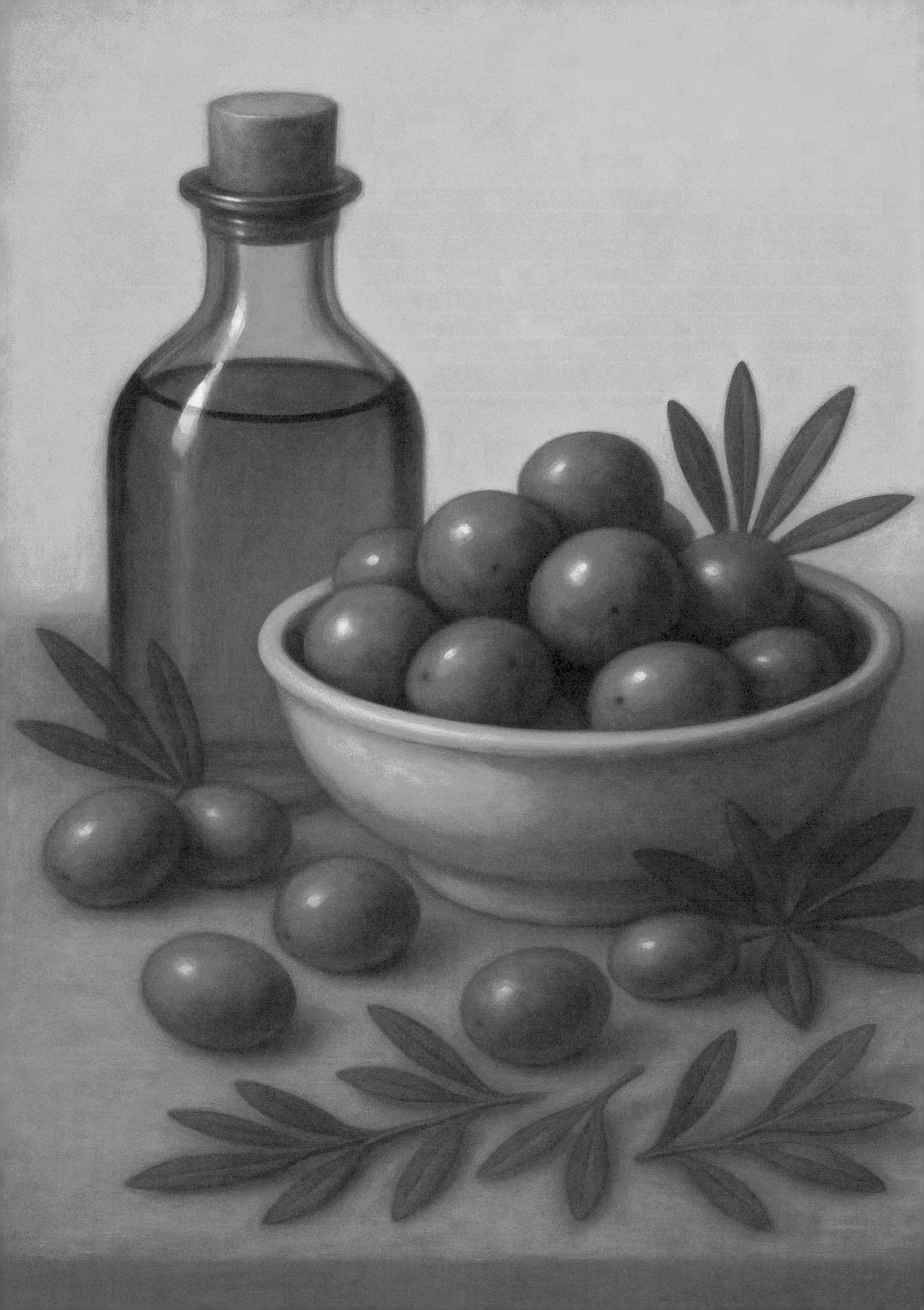

What Are Herb-Infused Olive Oils?

Herb-infused olive oils are flavorful creations made by steeping herbs in high-quality olive oil. They capture the aroma, flavor, and healing compounds of your herbs, offering a delicious way to elevate meals or body care.

These oils can be used in the kitchen or apothecary. They are delicious when used for dipping bread, drizzling on vegetables, dressing salads, or even as a base for cooking. They also work wonders as part of your skincare routine. Herb-infused oils can serve as a base for salves, hair masks, and skin moisturizers. While I personally prefer grape seed oil for skincare due to its nearly neutral scent, olive oil can also be used for both cooking and skin care purposes.

Note: For culinary oils, always use fully dried herbs to prevent spoilage. For topical oils, both fresh and dried herbs may be used, as long as proper care is taken. To be on the safe side, Wild Root Farm only uses dried herbs.

Basic Recipe for Herb-Infused Olive Oil

You'll need:

- 1 cup olive oil (cold-pressed, organic preferred)
- ¼–½ cup dried herbs
- A clean, dry glass jar with lid
- Cheesecloth for straining (optional)

Instructions:

1. **Add Herbs to a Clean Jar:**
   Fill the jar about ¼ to ½ full with dried herbs, depending on the strength you desire.
2. **Cover with Olive Oil:**
   Pour olive oil over the herbs, ensuring they are completely submerged.
3. **Infuse:**
   Seal the jar and place it in a warm, dark spot for 2–4 weeks. Shake gently every few days to help with the infusion process.
4. **Strain and Store:**
   After 2–4 weeks, strain the oil through cheesecloth, bottle it, and label.

Quick Infusion Method

For quicker results, you can gently heat the oil and herbs in a double boiler for 1–2 hours on low heat.

Storage Tips:

- Keep infused oils in a cool, dark place.
- For culinary oils: Use within 1–2 months. Refrigerate if unsure.
- For topical oils: Use within 6–12 months and always smell before use.

CULINARY INFUSED OLIVE OILS NOTES

Personal Experiences

Preparations Tried

Favorite Uses

Blends / Parings

Harvest Notes

Other thoughts

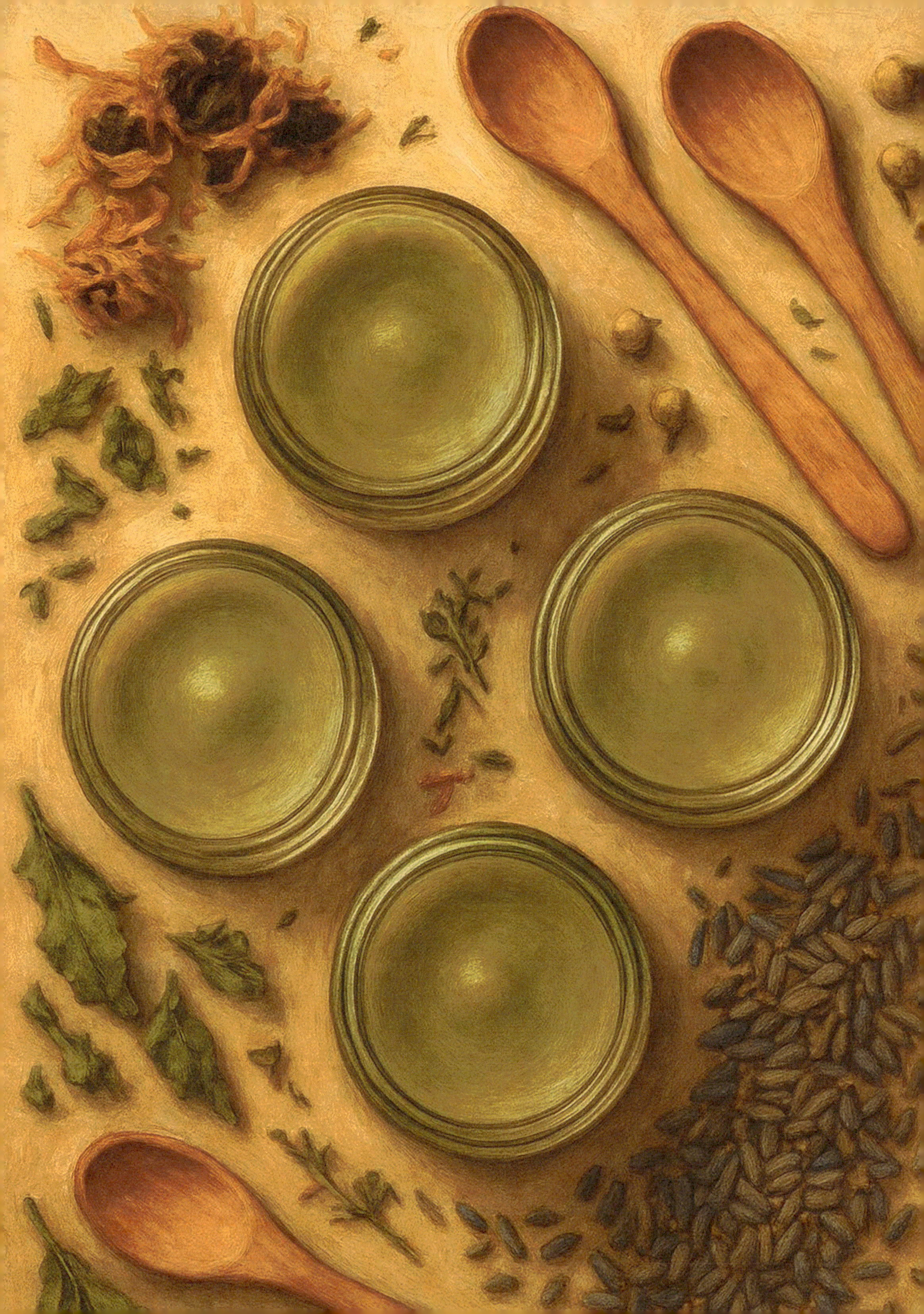

Topical Remedies

What Are Topical Remedies?

Topical remedies are plant-based preparations applied directly to the skin. They are designed to support the body from the outside in. These remedies can include simple herbal-infused oils, teas used as rinses, or salves. They don't need to be complicated—less is often more.

What Is an Infused Oil? (For Topical Use)

Herbal-infused oil is made by steeping dried herbs in a carrier oil to extract the plant's beneficial compounds, scent, and color. The result is a fragrant, nourishing oil that can be used for skin care, massage, salves, hair treatments, or even culinary use (depending on the oil and herb chosen).

Unlike essential oils, which are distilled and highly concentrated, infused oils are gentle, easy to make at home, and a staple in any herbal apothecary.

How to Make Herbal-Infused Oil

You'll Need

- Dried herbs (to prevent mold)
- A carrier oil (like olive, jojoba, almond, or coconut)
- A clean, dry glass jar with lid

Instructions

Option 1: Slow Solar Infusion (No-Heat Method)

1. **Fill a Clean, Dry Jar:**
   Add your dried herbs to a sterilized glass jar (fill about ½ to ¾ full with herbs).
2. **Cover With Oil:**
   Pour oil over the herbs until they're completely submerged. Use a clean skewer to release air bubbles.
3. **Infuse:**
   Cap tightly and place the jar in a sunny windowsill for 2–4 weeks. Shake gently every day.
4. **Strain:**
   After infusing, strain the oil through cheesecloth or a fine mesh strainer. Squeeze out every drop.
5. **Store:**
   Transfer to a dark glass bottle or jar. Label and store in a cool, dark place. Shelf-stable for 6–12 months.

Option 2: Quick Warm Infusion (Low Heat)

1. **Combine Herbs & Oil:**
   In a double boiler or heat-safe jar in a warm water bath, combine dried herbs and oil.
2. **Gently Heat:**
   Keep the temperature under 120°F (warm to the touch but never frying-hot). Infuse for 1–3 hours. Stir occasionally.
3. **Strain & Store:**
   Strain as above, bottle, and store in a cool, dark place.

Storage Tips:
• Keep in a cool, dark place.
• For culinary oils: Use within 1–2 months, and refrigerate if unsure.
• For topical oils: Use within 6–12 months and always smell before use.

What Is a Salve?

A salve is a thick, soothing ointment made by combining herbal-infused oils with beeswax (or a plant-based wax). It creates a semi-solid balm that's used topically to nourish, protect, and support the skin. Salves are one of the oldest forms of herbal medicine, offering targeted relief for everything from cuts and scrapes to sore muscles, dry skin, rashes, or chest congestion—depending on the herbs used.

Unlike creams or lotions, salves contain no water and have a long shelf life. They're ideal for making your herbal remedies portable, giftable, and easy to use on the go.

How to Make a Basic Herbal Salve

You'll Need

• Herbal-infused oil (see page 176)
• Beeswax (or candelilla wax for a vegan version)
• Optional: essential oils, vitamin E, or dried flowers for decoration

Basic Formula
• 1 cup infused oil
• ¼ cup beeswax pastilles (Use a little more for a firmer salve, less for a softer one.)

Instructions

1. **Melt Together:**
   In a double boiler, gently heat the infused oil and beeswax until fully melted.
2. **Add Extras:**
   Remove from heat and stir in essential oils (10–20 drops) or vitamin E if desired.
3. **Pour Into Jars:**
   Carefully pour into clean tins or glass jars.
4. **Let Set:**
   Allow to cool and solidify before sealing and labeling.

Tip: Test the texture by dropping a spoonful onto a cold plate. If it's too soft, add more beeswax; too firm, add more oil.

Can You Use Honeycomb Instead of Beeswax in a Salve?

Yes, but with care.
Honeycomb contains beeswax, but also traces of raw honey, pollen, and propolis—which are all beneficial but can complicate things if not handled properly. Therefore, I recommend doing this only if you are a seasoned user. If handled incorrectly, you might end up with a product you can't use, wasting both time and herbs.

Key Considerations:

1. **Purity**
   Raw honeycomb will melt unevenly and may leave behind sticky residues or moisture from the honey.
   • Moisture can cause spoilage or shorten the shelf life of your salve.

Tip: To use honeycomb safely, gently render it into pure beeswax first.

How to Render Beeswax from Honeycomb:

1. Break up the comb into small pieces.
2. Place in a double boiler with just enough water to prevent scorching.
3. Gently heat until the wax melts and separates from the honey and debris.
4. Strain through cheesecloth into a mold or jar and let cool.
5. Once solid, the clean beeswax can be used in salves like normal!

Final Verdict

• Raw honeycomb = not ideal directly in a salve
• Rendered beeswax = yes, absolutely

Herbal Topical Rinse

Ingredients:

• 1–2 tablespoons dried herb (or 2–4 tablespoons fresh)
• 2 cups boiling water

Optional: Add 1 tablespoon apple cider vinegar for hair/scalp support or skin pH balance.

Instructions:

1. **Steep the Herbs:**
   Place herbs in a heat-safe jar or bowl. Pour 2 cups boiling water over them. Cover and steep for 15–30 minutes (or longer for stronger rinses).
2. **Strain & Cool:**
   Strain out herbs with cheesecloth or a fine strainer. Allow the liquid to cool to room temperature.
3. **Use Immediately:**
   Use within 24 hours, or refrigerate and use within 3 days. Do not store long-term unless preserved.

How to Use

Hair Rinse (for shine, scalp health)
After shampooing, pour herbal rinse over hair and massage into scalp. Leave on or rinse lightly.

Facial Rinse (for breakouts or irritation)
Splash over clean skin or apply with a cloth. Calendula, chamomile, sage, or rosemary are ideal.

Foot or Body Soak (for muscle tension or odor)
Add to a warm basin or bath. Lavender, spearmint, or thyme are great here.

Skin Rinse or Compress (for minor cuts, eczema, or bug bites)
Soak a clean cloth in the rinse and apply as a warm or cool compress to the skin.

Herb Suggestions

• **Calendula or chamomile** – soothe skin, reduce inflammation
• **Lavender or lemon balm** – calm itching, promote healing
• **Sage or rosemary** – cleanse oily scalp, help dandruff
• **Holy basil or nettle** – tone skin, nourish follicles
• **Spearmint or thyme** – deodorize, refresh tired feet

TOPICAL REMEDIES NOTES

Personal Experiences

Preparations Tried

Favorite Uses

Blends / Parings

Harvest Notes

Other thoughts

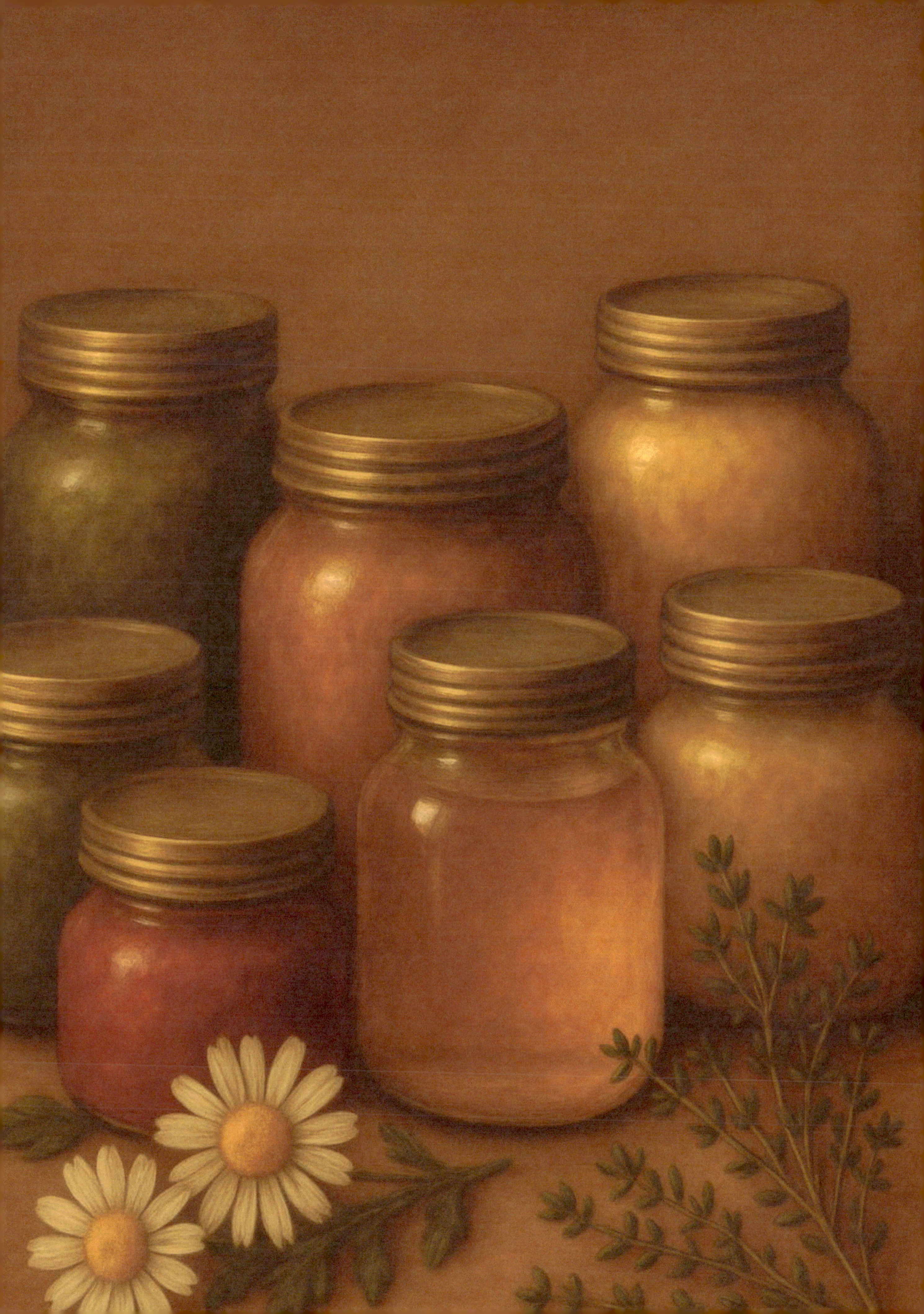

What Is a Sugar Scrub?

Sugar scrubs are simple, all-natural exfoliants. Typically made from sugar blended with oils, herbs, and often aromatic ingredients like essential oils or dried flowers, these scrubs gently polish away dead skin cells. They leave your skin soft, glowing, and deeply moisturized.

Because sugar is a natural humectant (it draws moisture to the skin), sugar scrubs are both exfoliating and hydrating. They're perfect for dry hands, rough elbows, tired feet, or full-body pampering.

How to Make a Simple Herbal Sugar Scrub

You'll Need

- Natural sugar (white for fine scrubs, brown for coarser)
- A carrier oil (like coconut, sweet almond, or olive oil)
- Optional: dried herbs, flower petals, essential oils, or citrus zest

Basic Formula

- 1 cup sugar
- ½ cup oil (adjust to desired texture)
- Optional add-ins: 1–2 tsp dried herb, 5–10 drops essential oil, 1 tsp citrus zest

Instructions

1. **Mix Ingredients:**
   Combine sugar and oil in a bowl until evenly blended.
2. **Add Extras:**
   Stir in herbs, essential oils, or other add-ins.
3. **Jar It Up:**
   Spoon into a clean glass jar with a lid. Label and store in a cool spot.
4. **To Use:**
   Massage gently onto damp skin in circular motions. Rinse with warm water and pat dry.

BATH & BODY NOTES

Personal Experiences

Preparations Tried

Favorite Uses

Blends / Parings

Harvest Notes

Other thoughts

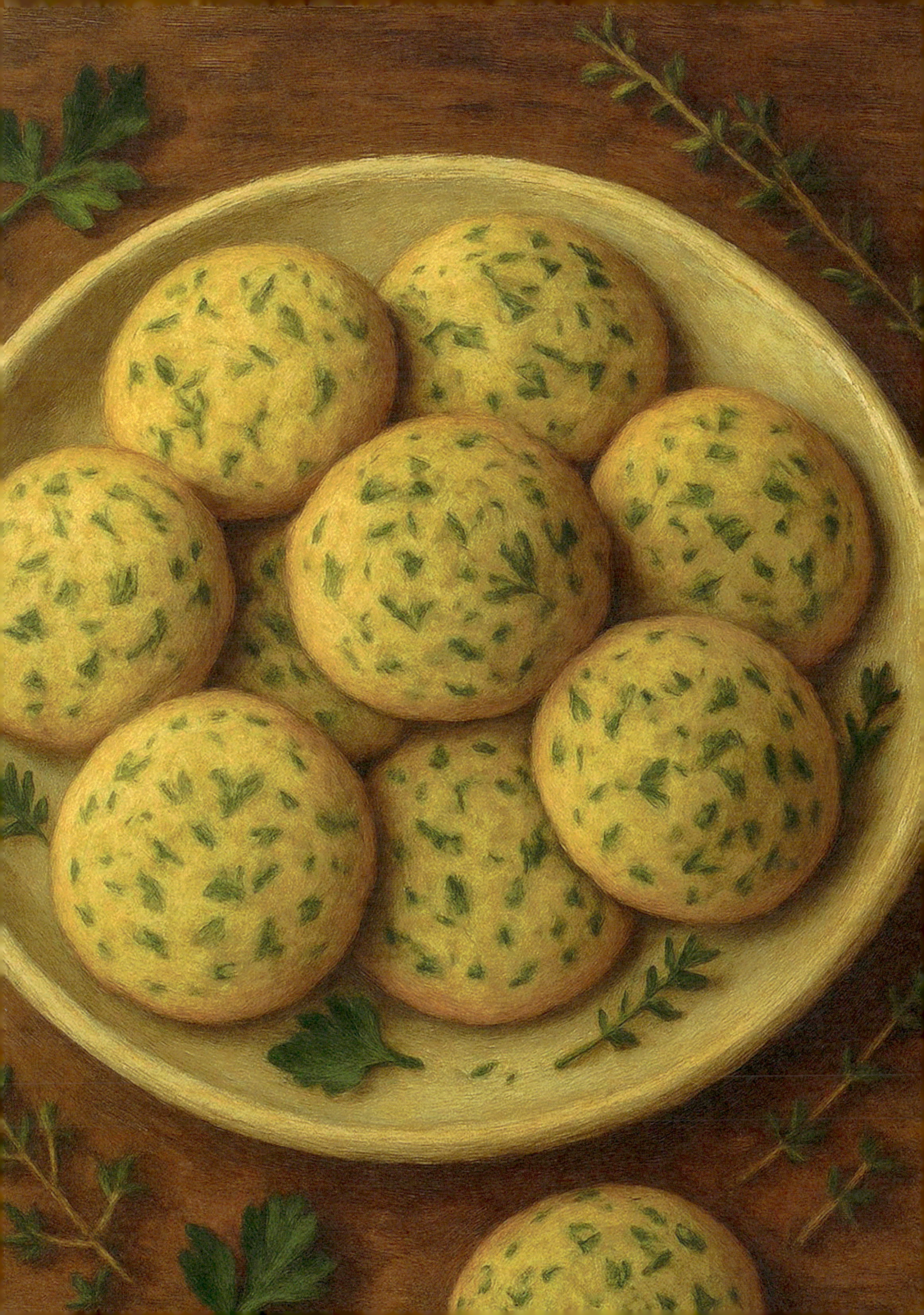

Herbal Magic in Every Bite

Shortbread dough is the perfect blank canvas for herbs like:

- **Lavender** – calming and floral
- **Rosemary** – earthy and unexpected
- **Lemon Balm or Thyme** – bright and citrusy
- **Mint or Holy Basil** – refreshing and uplifting
- **Chamomile** – dreamy and sweet

You can also roll the dough in crushed dried herbs, decorate with pressed edible flowers, or drizzle with infused honey.

Basic Herbal Shortbread Bite Formula

Ingredients

- 1 cup butter, softened
- ½ cup powdered sugar
- 2 cups flour
- 1–2 tablespoons finely chopped fresh herbs (or 1 tsp dried)
- Pinch of salt and optional citrus zest or vanilla

Instructions

1. **Cream butter and sugar** until light and fluffy.
2. **Add herbs** and dry ingredients and mix into a soft dough.
3. **Roll into a log**, chill, then slice into coins or cut into small shapes.
4. **Bake** at 325°F for 12–15 minutes, until edges are lightly golden. Cool and enjoy!

Tip: These cookies pair beautifully with herbal tea—try matching herb to tea for a full-circle garden treat!

Basic Herbal Cracker Formula

Ingredients

- 1 cup flour (all-purpose, whole wheat, or gluten-free)
- 2–3 tablespoons olive oil or melted butter
- ¼ cup water (as needed)
- 1–2 tablespoons finely chopped herbs
- Optional: salt, seeds, garlic powder, nutritional yeast, or cheese

Instructions

1. Preheat oven to 375°F.
2. **In a bowl**, combine flour, herbs, and any seasonings.
3. **Add oil** and mix, then slowly stir in water until a dough forms.
4. **Roll thinly** between two pieces of parchment paper.
5. **Cut into shapes** (squares, rounds, or rustic strips) and place on a baking sheet.
6. **Bake** for 12–15 minutes, until golden and crisp. Cool before storing.

Tip: Store in an airtight jar or tin for up to a week or freeze dough to bake later. Brush with olive oil before baking for extra flavor.

Peppermint Herbal Chocolate

Cool. Comforting. A melt-in-your-mouth herbal delight.

Ingredients

• 1 cup dark chocolate chips or chopped chocolate (70% or higher)
• 1–2 teaspoons dried peppermint leaves (or ½ tsp peppermint extract)
• Optional: crushed candy cane, cacao nibs, or a pinch of sea salt

Directions

1. **Melt the Chocolate:**
   In a heatproof bowl, gently melt chocolate over a double boiler or in short bursts in the microwave, stirring often.
2. **Infuse with Peppermint:**
   If using dried peppermint:
   - Stir it directly into the melted chocolate and let steep for 5–10 minutes.
   - Strain if desired, or leave the herb in for texture and extra flavor.
     If using peppermint extract:
   - Add it once the chocolate is fully melted and smooth. Stir well.
3. **Pour and Set:**
   Pour the chocolate into molds, a lined tray, or spoon into small discs. Sprinkle with crushed peppermint candy or sea salt if desired.
4. **Cool:**
   Let set at room temperature or refrigerate until firm. Store in a cool, dry place.

Tip: A perfect way to turn a powerful digestive herb into a soothing treat. Great after meals, as a gift, or for a moment of mindful indulgence.

Herb-Infused Jelly

A sweet way to preserve the magic of herbs. It's also a great way to get finicky eaters to get a dose of herbal medicine. Herbal jellies capture both the flavor and healing energy of your garden in a spoonful. Use floral, minty, or citrusy herbs to create a jelly that's delicious on toast, paired with cheese, or stirred into tea.

Ingredients

- 2 cups strong herbal infusion (see below)
- 1 tablespoon lemon juice (adds acidity & preserves color)
- 1 box (1.75 oz) powdered pectin
- 2½ cups sugar

Great herbs for jelly: lemon balm, rose petals, lavender, mint, thyme, holy basil, red clover.

Instructions

1. **Make the Herbal Infusion**
   Steep ½–1 cup dried herbs (or 1–2 cups fresh) in 2½ cups boiling water for 20–30 minutes. Strain and measure 2 cups of strong tea.
2. **Prepare Your Workspace**
   Sterilize jars and lids. Set up a clean, heat-safe surface and have a ladle, funnel, and jars ready.
3. **Cook the Jelly**
   - In a saucepan, combine the herbal tea and lemon juice.
   - Sprinkle in the powdered pectin and stir well.
   - Bring the mixture to a boil over medium-high heat.
4. **Add the Sugar**
   - Stir in the sugar all at once. Return to a rolling boil, stirring constantly.
   - Boil hard for 1–2 minutes until jelly thickens slightly (use the spoon test or thermometer—220°F).
5. **Jar and Seal**
   - Remove from heat and skim any foam.
   - Ladle jelly into hot jars, leaving ¼-inch headspace.
   - Wipe rims, apply lids, and process in a hot water bath for 10 minutes (if storing shelf-stable).

TREATS & SNACK NOTES

Personal Experiences

Preparations Tried

Favorite Uses

Blends / Parings

Harvest Notes

Other thoughts

Herbal Pillow Sachets

Pillow sachets are small fabric bundles filled with dried herbs to promote rest, relaxation, and gentle dreams. Place one near your pillow, tuck it into drawers, or gift them as bundles of calm.

What You'll Need

- ¼ to ½ cup dried herbs of choice (lavender, chamomile, lemon balm, rosemary, or mint)
- Small fabric squares (cotton, linen, or muslin work best)
- Needle & thread, or a sewing machine
- Optional: ribbon, lace, or drawstring bags

Instructions

1. **Choose Your Herbs**
   Select dried herbs based on their properties:
   • Lavender & chamomile — promote calm and sleep
   • Rosemary & lemon balm — soothe the heart
   • Mint or holy basil — gently refresh and uplift
   You may blend several herbs or use a single star herb.
2. **Make Your Sachet**
   Cut two small fabric squares (around 4" x 4"). Place them right sides together, and stitch around the edges, leaving a small opening. Turn the pouch right side out.
3. **Fill with Herbs**
   Spoon in ¼–½ cup of dried herbs. Do not overpack—you want the pouch to remain soft and breathable.
4. **Close the Sachet**
   Sew the opening closed by hand or machine. Optionally, decorate with ribbon, buttons, or lace.
   Alternative: Use pre-made muslin drawstring bags for a no-sew option—perfect for bulk making or gifts.

Tips for Use
- Keep near your pillow or in your linen drawer
- Refresh scent by gently squeezing the sachet
- Replace herbs every 3–6 months as scent fades

Summer Simmer Pots

Summer simmer pots are warm-weather versions of traditional stovetop potpourri, designed to fill your home with light, herbal, and uplifting scents that reflect the season of sunshine and bloom. Rather than the heavy spices of winter, summer pots focus on fresh herbs, citrus, florals, and soft garden notes. Using herbs you've grown or gathered, these simmer pots can set a calming mood, freshen the air, and invite a sense of ritual and gratitude for the season. Pick a blend based on your mood or intention and simmer gently in a pot of water (or a slow cooker). Let the steam work its magic.

Uplifting & Joyful

- Lemon balm – bright and citrusy
- Calendula petals – cheerful and golden
- Spearmint – fresh and sweet
- Optional: lemon slices, vanilla bean

Perfect for warm afternoons and open windows.

Calm & Clear
- Chamomile – relaxing and apple-scented
- Holy basil (Tulsi) – peaceful and grounding
- Optional: orange peel, rosemary

Ideal for early mornings or unwinding after a busy day.

Clean & Earthy
- Thyme – crisp and clarifying
- Sage – clearing and sacred
- Rosemary – purifying and invigorating
- Optional: green apple slices, eucalyptus leaves

Use during house cleaning or energetic reset days.

Wild Garden Blend
- Nettle – mineral-rich, subtle earth scent
- Holy basil – uplifting but grounding
- Calendula + mint – harmony in a pot
- Optional: fresh herbs on the turn, a splash of berry juice

A celebration of your herb garden at peak summer.

Instructions

1. Fill a small pot or slow cooker halfway with water.
2. Add herbs (fresh or dried), fruit slices, or petals.
3. Simmer uncovered on low. Refill water as needed.
4. Let the scent carry through your space.

Tip: Save stems, petals, and leftover herbs in the freezer for easy simmer pot blends later.

What Is an Herbal Room Spray?

An herbal room spray is a natural, plant-based mist made with distilled water, alcohol, and essential oils or herbal extracts. It's used to freshen the air, shift the mood, or energetically cleanse a space—without synthetic fragrances or chemicals. Room sprays are one of the easiest ways to bring the aroma and energy of herbs into your home. Depending on the herbs used, they can be calming, uplifting, grounding, or purifying.

How to Make an Herbal Room Spray

You'll need:

- 2 oz glass spray bottle
- 1–2 teaspoons witch hazel or high-proof alcohol (helps preserve and disperse oils)
- Herbal tea

Instructions

1. **Fill the Bottle:** Add witch hazel or alcohol to the bottom of the bottle.
2. **Add Herbal Tea:** Choose herbs based on mood or purpose.
3. **Shake Well:** Always shake before each use, as oils naturally separate.

Tip: Label your blend with the date and store out of direct sunlight. Best used within 2–3 months for peak freshness.

HOME USES NOTES

Personal Experiences

Preparations Tried

Favorite Uses

Blends / Parings

Harvest Notes

Other thoughts

10 HERBS EVERYONE SHOULD GROW

GARDEN PLANNER

January

- Lemon Balm: Check overwintered plants; start indoors if zone-appropriate.
- Chamomile: Plan seed order; sow indoors in warm zones.
- Calendula: Order seeds; prepare pots or trays for February start.
- Tulsi: Only grow indoors now; start seeds in warmth + light.
- Yarrow: Divide roots if ground isn't frozen; prep indoor starts.
- Nettle: Plan where to grow it away from foot traffic!
- Rosemary: Bring potted plants indoors; avoid overwatering.
- Thyme: Trim leggy growth on overwintered plants indoors.
- Peppermint: Check for rootbound pots; propagate cuttings indoors.
- Echinacea: Order seeds; stratify now for spring planting.

February

- Lemon Balm: Start seeds indoors if early spring zone.
- Chamomile: Begin indoor sowing of German chamomile.
- Calendula: Sow indoors or cold-frame start in mild zones.
- Tulsi: Sow indoors on heat mat. Light essential.
- Yarrow: Indoor seed starts; prep garden spot.
- Nettle: Cold-stratify seeds for better germination.
- Rosemary: Prune lightly; start new cuttings.
- Thyme: Start seeds indoors or repot if needed.
- Peppermint: Keep in light; divide indoor pots.
- Echinacea: Finish cold-stratifying seeds.

March

- Lemon Balm: Transplant indoors starts to larger pots.
- Chamomile: Harden off starts in warmer zones.
- Calendula: Sow directly outside in mild climates.
- Tulsi: Transplant seedlings into larger pots.
- Yarrow: Sow outdoors or continue indoors.
- Nettle: Sow seeds outdoors if ground workable.
- Rosemary: Move pots outside on warm days.
- Thyme: Begin outdoor sowing in mild climates.
- Peppermint: Take cuttings or divide roots.
- Echinacea: Sow seeds outdoors in prepared bed..

April

- Lemon Balm: Transplant outdoors; mulch well.
- Chamomile: Sow directly if not started.
- Calendula: Sow more for staggered bloom.
- Tulsi: Keep inside unless consistently warm.
- Yarrow: Plant seedlings or divided roots.
- Nettle: Weed around nettle, give space.
- Rosemary: Harden off potted plants.
- Thyme: Plant out in garden beds.
- Peppermint: Plant into containers or beds.
- Echinacea: Thin or transplant seedlings.

May

- Lemon Balm: Begin light harvest of young leaves.
- Chamomile: Blossoms appear—begin harvest.
- Calendula: First blooms—start drying.
- Tulsi: Harden off and plant outside.
- Yarrow: Watch for first flowering shoots.
- Nettle: Cut for first spring flush.
- Rosemary: Feed with organic compost.
- Thyme: Begin pruning for shape + harvest.
- Peppermint: Pinch tips for bushier growth.
- Echinacea: Keep weeds away, water deeply.

June

- Lemon Balm: Harvest before flowering.
- Chamomile: Frequent flower picking = more blooms.
- Calendula: Daily deadheading.
- Tulsi: Pinch off flower buds for more leaves.
- Yarrow: Harvest flowering tops.
- Nettle: Second harvest before flowers.
- Rosemary: Trim for drying, don't overdo.
- Thyme: Harvest right before bloom for potency.
- Peppermint: Harvest early morning.
- Echinacea: Watch for first blooms.

July

- Lemon Balm: Harvest again if regrown.
- Chamomile: Pick daily if blooming.
- Calendula: Keep deadheading!
- Tulsi: Harvest leaves, pinch flower tops.
- Yarrow: Dry cuttings; divide if needed.
- Nettle: Let flower or cut for compost.
- Rosemary: Water deeply in heat.
- Thyme: Prune lightly after bloom.
- Peppermint: Cut back to promote new growth.
- Echinacea: Enjoy blooms; avoid cutting all (for pollinators).

August

- Lemon Balm: Collect seeds or allow to go to seed.
- Chamomile: Gather seeds if faded.
- Calendula: Continue deadheading.
- Tulsi: Harvest before full flowering.
- Yarrow: Save seeds or divide roots.
- Nettle: Cut for fall regrowth or let reseed.
- Rosemary: Light prune to shape.
- Thyme: Harvest for drying.
- Peppermint: Cut back to refresh plant.
- Echinacea: Leave seed heads for pollinators.

September

- Lemon Balm: Final harvest; dry leaves.
- Chamomile: Save seeds from mature flowers.
- Calendula: Collect seeds; compost old stems.
- Tulsi: Final harvest before cooler nights.
- Yarrow: Divide and replant if needed.
- Nettle: Cut to soil level; leave roots.
- Rosemary: Pot up to bring indoors in cold zones.
- Thyme: Final trimming.
- Peppermint: Dig and divide if crowded.
- Echinacea: Leave for fall interest + wildlife.

October

- Lemon Balm: Mulch root zone for winter.
- Chamomile: Remove dead growth.
- Calendula: Sow fall crop in warm zones.
- Tulsi: Harvest roots if growing medicinally.
- Yarrow: Mulch if in cold zone.
- Nettle: Add to compost or fall tea blends.
- Rosemary: Bring indoors (if zone requires).
- Thyme: Mulch and clean up around plant.
- Peppermint: Cut down, mulch.
- Echinacea: Leave standing for birds.

November

- Lemon Balm: Dormant; protect roots.
- Chamomile: Enjoy dried tea stash.
- Calendula: Dry remaining flowers if found.
- Tulsi: Use dried leaves for tea blends.
- Yarrow: Resting. Label dried bundles.
- Nettle: Use dried for nourishing infusions.
- Rosemary: Prune if moving indoors.
- Thyme: Use fresh sparingly; enjoy dried.
- Peppermint: Use in winter tonics.
- Echinacea: Let overwinter for seed + structure.

December

- Lemon Balm: Check overwintering mulch.
- Chamomile: Plan tea blends, organize seeds.
- Calendula: Plan for spring sowing.
- Tulsi: Review harvest notes + prep seeds.
- Yarrow: Organize herbal blends.
- Nettle: Steep dried leaves for winter tonic.
- Rosemary: Mist indoor plant, avoid drafts.
- Thyme: Use fresh if available.
- Peppermint: Add to winter salves + teas.
- Echinacea: Enjoy dried root or tincture making.

Made in United States
Troutdale, OR
04/27/2026

48797792R00126